201 Tips to Control High Blood Pressure

Dr. Bimal Chhajer, MD

DIAMOND BOOKS

Publisher : **Diamond Pocket Books (P) Ltd.**
X-30, Okhla Industrial Area, Phase-II
New Delhi-110020
Phone : 011-40712200
E-mail : sales@dpb.in
Website : www.diamondbook.in

---

201 Tips to Control High Blood Pressure

By - *Dr. Bimal Chhajer, MD*

Introduction

High Blood Pressure is known as Hypertension in medical community- it is one of the most important silent killers. Presently it is estimated that India has 5 crore patients suffering from Hypertension. An increase of blood pressure from 120/80 mmHg to 150/100 mmHg can reduce our lifespan by 11.5 years. High blood pressure is also known to increase risks of paralysis(Stroke) by 20 percent and coronary heart disease(blockage in the arteries of heart) by 15 percent.

There are many causes of HT. It may be caused by overweight, wrong food habits (especially high salt diet, low intake of potassium and calcium and high fat diet), stress or psychosocial factors, lack of physical activity and so on. Smoking and high blood pressure if combined together, increase the chances of heart attack much more. But it is assumed that, psychological stress is the most important cause of high Blood Pressure and contributes 50% to the cause of this disease.

Hypertension is one of the major killer diseases and yet it damages silently. In case of the heart, it leads to blockages, heart attacks, enlargement of the heart and heart failures. It also leads to stroke or paralysis, sudden unconsciousness(TIA), brain damage and loss of memory. In the Eye - it can lead to bleeding and complete blindness. It can not only lead to kidney damage but also damage to many other organs.

The cause of concern is that most of the high blood pressure cases go undetected because it often does not have any symptoms. A doctor mostly detects it during a casual check-up. Even after the diagnosis - a large number of high BP patients do not take treatment or remain inadequately treated. There is a saying "Out of all the patients of hypertension, 50% go undetected, out of those who get detected, 50% do not take treatment and out of those who take treatment, 50% are not adequately treated."

The silver lining or the good message is that high blood pressure can be measured very easily and non-invasively within few seconds. The instrument to measure blood pressure is not expensive, is easy to use and can be used with very little training. Almost 60% of the blood pressure patients can be treated with lifestyle changes only and rest of the 40% can be well managed with a combination of lifestyle and drugs. But all of them are manageable. Even in the absence of lifestyle changes, drugs can take care for short periods.

Life today is full of tensions and pressures. High Blood Pressure has started even in young age group, both in males and females. Every individual living under pressure or excessive stress or having a sedentary lifestyle and every executive above the age of 25 must get their blood pressure checked up regularly. Remember that the normal blood pressure is 120/80 mmHg and not above this. In case of three consective readings more than 130/85 mmHg, the treatment must be started.

In this book, which is mainly meant for the patients with High Blood Pressure, I am going to explain the cause and effect of High Blood Pressure on our body; explain what we can do to take care of this common but fatal disease. I am going to emphasize more on non drug treatment of high BP so that continuous intake of tablets to control BP is not required for a long period. This treatment will include advice to cut down stress or tension, lifestyle changes, know how about diet and cooking food, weight reduction tips, yoga, exercise and walking.

This book is very important because crores of High Blood Pressure patients in India do not have any direct access to knowledge about what all they can do to take care of their Blood Pressure. Most of the physicians do not have time to explain these factors or train the high BP patients. The cardiologists are not at all interested in patients who just want to control high BP. They would like to treat patients who need Bypass Surgery or Angioplasty or has a heart attack. The net result is that most of the high BP Patients do not get proper treatment or keep on taking only medicines. This book will give a complete knowledge which is usable by the high BP patients and solve their queries about what to do and what not to do.

About the Author

Dr. Bimal Chhajer, MD is the pioneering cardiologist who has developed 'SAAOL Heart Program', one of the most popular non-invasive heart care and treatment programs in India. Dr. Chhajer was born in 1961 in a Jain family. He hails from Rajasthan but has grown up in Kolkata. He passed his MBBS from R.G. Kar Medical College, Kolkata in 1986. He materialized the concept of bringing all the possible useful items together, be it from Science or Art to treat heart patients. His insight has helped thousands of patients to cure themselves without going for Bypass Surgery or Angioplasty, without any risk.

At the age of 25 years he left Kolkata for Delhi, where he started working in the Cardiology department in Dr. Ram Manohar Lohia Hospital, New Delhi. He then completed his MD from King George's Medical College, Lucknow where he took up a research study to treat heart patients non-invasively.

He has worked as an Assistant Professor at the All India Institute of Medical Sciences (AIIMS) and carried out his research work at AIIMS for six years when he developed the program. He also got training in Yoga Therapy.He also represented AIIMS at the Eleventh Antartica Expedition from India.

Dr. Chhajer, during this period also got trained by Dr. Dean Ornish, who pioneered the lifestyle treatment in USA and proved Reversal of heart Disease by his Lifestyle heart Trial to the medical science. Dr. Chhajer opened various clinics in Mumbai, Kolkata, Jaipur, Jodhpur, Bangalore and Hyderabad. His head office is situated in Vikram Vihar, Lajpat Nagar, New Delhi.

He has not only lectured all over India and the world but has also been in the field of cardiology for more than 15 years. He is also the author of many books.

1. Reversal of Heart Disease in Five Easy Steps
2. Food for Reversing Heart Disease
3. Hriday Rog Se Mukti
4. Understanding Heart Disease
5. Hriday Rog Samanya Jankari

6. Zero Oil Cook Book (Hindi and English)
7. Zero Oil Sweet Book (Hindi and English)
8. Zero Oil Namkeen Book (Hindi and English)
9. Zero Oil South Indian Cook Book (Hindi and English)
10. 201 Diet Tips For Heart Patients (Hindi and English)
11. A Complete Guide to Stress Management
12. A Complete Meal without Oil. (Hindi and English)
13. 201 Tips for Losing Weight
14. 201 Tips for Diabetes Patients
15. Zero Oil 151 Snacks
16. Health in Your Hand (12 books Series on different diseases)
17. Learn how to Reverse Heart Disease?
18. A Complete Guide Managing Stress.

Today his brainchild "Saaol Heart Program" is a widely accepted treatment program for Reversing Heart Disease - where in addition to the allopathic medicines patients are taught Yoga, Meditation, Zero Oil cooking, Stress Management, Exercises and Medical Knowledge.

He also brings out a monthly journal 'Saaol Times' covering a wide range of heart related topics. Now 'Saaol Samachar' (Hindi) is also available. More than 1000 articles have been written in magazines and newspapers about him and SAAOL Heart Program. He has regularly appeared in TV programs, news talks. He has brought out many VCDs and DVDs on every health topic that is possible.

Dr. Chhajer organised the First International Conference, in conjunction with AIIMS on 'Life Style and Heart' in 1995 at India Habitat Centre, New Delhi and 2nd International Conference on 'Life Style and Health' in November 1999, at the same venue.

Dr. Chhajer has also launched day course for Arthritis, Asthma, Diabetes and Obesity., which are most common modern day afflictions.

Dr. Bimal Chhajer has till now treated more than 12000 heart patients and helped them to avoid heart attack, Bypass Surgery and Angioplasty. He has treated India's Ex-President Late Shree Shankar Dayaljee Sharma. The Present President of India, Honourable Mrs. Pratibha D. Patil and her husband has also taken a three days' heart care training from Dr. Chhajer. Dr. Chhajer has been awarded many times including "Rajeev Gandhi Rastriya Ekta Award".

SAAOL HEART PROGRAM

The SAAOL Heart Program is an extensive three days training program where a group of heart patients stay together to learn the "science and art of living". Under the guidance of doctors, dieticians, yoga experts and trainers they are taught medical know how about lifestyle related diseases and heart disease. This program will help one to get rid of Blood pressure and prevent/reverse Heart disease. The patients along with their spouses learn the perfect art of heart care.

This camp is organized in all the metros. In Delhi, it is held every month and every three months in rest of the metros (Kolkata, Bangalore & Mumbai). By joining this camp you can avoid Bypass surgery, Angioplasty, Angiography and Heart attack.

For more details and free booklet write to:

Saaol's Office:

North Zone : Delhi (Head Office)
SAAOL Heart Center
14/84-85, Vikram Vihar, Lajpat Nagar IV, New Delhi - 110024
Ph. : 011-26235168, 26283098, 26211908, 65093130
Fax : 26212016
E-mail : info@saaol.com, website : www.saaol.com
South Delhi: 78, National Park, New Delhi
Tel: 011-65178530.

East Delhi: Saaol Heart Center
1, Surya Niketan, Vikas Marg Ext., Delhi- 92
Tel.: 011-22377358, 22377359

North Delhi: Saaol Heart Center
B-177, Lok Vihar, Pitampura, Delhi-34
Tel: 011-27352023, 65158202

Jaipur Center: Saaol Heart Center
21-D-1, Barwada House Colony
(Near Ajmer Pulia) Ajmer Road, Jaipur-302006
Tel: 0141-4007141, 2220037 Mobile: 9829060442.
Email: saaolheartcenter@yahoo.com

Jodhpur Center: Suncity Heart Care Center
Paota, Jodhpur (Rajsthan)
Tel: 0291-2545455, 2546455

South Zone : Bangalore
Mr. Jaikar/ Mrs. Smita
No. 16, 17th "A" Cross, Bhuvaneswari Nagar,
Opp. Coffee Board Layout Play Ground, Bangalore-560024
Mobile : 9343736554, Ph: 64524482
E-mail : ssprasaad@yahoo.com

Chennai Office: Mr. Kamal Chhajer
C/o Jeans Park India Pvt. Ltd, 566, Anna Salai, Chennai- 600018
Ph.: 044-22260209, Mobile: 93809-22206

Hyderabad Office: Saaol Heart Center
3-6-147/2, Street No.17, Himayat Nagar,
(Besides Vasu Medical Hall, Opp. HDFC Bank)
Himayat Nagar, Hyderabad- 500029
Ph.: 092462-28104

West Zone : Saaol Heart Center, Mumbai
Ms. Sudha/ Mr. Gaurav Agarwal
Sakeel Mansion, Ground Floor Flat No.2, Juhu Tara Road,
Opp. JW Marriott Hotel, Mumbai- 49
Ph.: 022-32094948, Mobile: 9819809068

East Zone : Kolkata
Mr. Praveen
65/4A, Flat No.: 1A, Sarat Bose Road, Kolkata-25
Ph.: 033-32930329, 24545981, Mob.: 9330870713.

Contents

CHAPTER-1

Understanding Blood Pressure (BP) and Hypertension (HT)

1. Working of the Cardiovascular System ----- 19
   - Cardiovascular System ----- 19
   - What is High BP or Hypertension? ----- 20
   - Need for Blood Pressure ----- 20
   - The Organs that control blood pressure ----- 21
2. Causes or Risk factors for High Blood Pressure ----- 23
   - Non Modifiable risk factors ----- 23
   - Modifiable risk factors ----- 23
   - Does Tension or stress lead to High Blood Pressure? ----- 24
3. Common Knowledge about High Blood Pressure ----- 26
   - What is normal BP or High BP? ----- 26
   - How is High BP diagnosed? ----- 27
   - What are the symptoms of High BP? ----- 27
4. - Primary (Essential) Hypertension ----- 29
   - Secondary Hypertension ----- 30

CHAPTER-2

Blood Pressure Measurement ----- 33

- General Technique ----- 33
- Understanding the Technique of Measurement of BP ----- 34
- Types of Blood Pressure Equipments ----- 34
- Do's and Don'ts about BP measurements ----- 35

CHAPTER-3

Plan of Treatment of High Blood Pressure ----- 36

CHAPTER-4

Diet for Treatment of High Blood Pressure ----- 40

- High salt intake and hypertension ----- 40

- Salt sensitivity ----- 41
- Dash Diet ----- 41
- Diet low in cholesterol and fats ----- 42
- Diet for Reduction of weight ----- 43
- Diet for High fiber and Anti Oxidants ----- 48

CHAPTER-5

Stress management to control High Blood Pressure ---- 49

- Rational and Emotional Brain ----- 50
- Understanding Stress and its effects on our life ----- 50
- How to identify a stressed person? ----- 51
- The production of Stress ----- 54
- Handling of External Factors ----- 55
- Mindset and its handling ----- 59
- Pressures of Life ----- 61
- Balancing the stress sectors of life ----- 62
- Communication skill ----- 66
- Releasing and Managing Stress ----- 67
- Yoga for Stress Management ----- 69
- Time Management ----- 71

CHAPTER-6

Yoga for High Blood Pressure Patients ---- 72

- Introduction ----- 72
- Definition ----- 72
- Eight steps of Yoga ----- 73
- Meditation ----- 73
- Scientific effects of Yoga & Meditation on the body ----- 75
- Rules and regulations ----- 76
- The Yogic diet ----- 77
- Health Rejuvenating Exercises (HRE) ----- 78
- Yoga Asana for lowering high BP ----- 82
- Kayotsarga ----- 85
- Preksha meditation ----- 87
- Anupreksha and moral code ----- 89

CHAPTER-7

Habits to change ----- 90

- Stop Smoking
- Avoid Alcohol
- Avoid Coffee & Tea
- Read Food lebels
- Sleep adequately
- Increase Physical Activity

CHAPTER-8

Walking and Exercise for High Blood Pressure Patients ---- 93

CHAPTER-9

Medicines for Treatment of High Blood Pressure ----- 95

- Introduction ----- 95
- Advantages of Allopathic medicines ----- 96
- Monitoring BP during treatment ----- 97
- Broad groups of BP Medicines ----- 99
- Side effects of Medicines ---- 103
- Some common points on High BP Medicines ---- 103
- Treatment Chart ---- 105

CHAPTER-10

Complications of High Blood Pressure ---- 106

CHAPTER-11

Hypertension during Pregnancy ---- 108

CHAPTER-12

201 Questions or Tips on High Blood Pressure --- 109

- ***General Questions:***

1. What is Blood Pressure? Why do we need it? ---- 109
2. What is the normal BP? ---- 109
3. What is Hypertension? ---- 109
4. What is the latest figure for normal Blood Pressure? ---- 109
5. What is "mmHg"? ---- 110
6. What is systolic Blood Pressure? ---- 110
7. What is diastolic Blood Pressure? ---- 110
8. How is Blood Pressure measured? ---- 110

9. What is meant by mean Blood Pressure? ---- 111
10. Does Blood Pressure differ according to Age? ---- 111
11. What happens in low BP? ---- 111
12. How to diagnose low BP? ---- 111
13. What are the grades of HT? ---- 111
14. Which BP is more important – Systolic or diastolic? ---- 112
15. What is labile HT? ---- 112
16. What is Pre Hypertension? ---- 112
17. What is JNC? On what basis do they change the grading of HT? ---- 112
18. Many doctors still believe BP of 140/90 mmHg is normal. Is it OK.? ---- 112
19. There was a dictum that systolic BP is age+100. Is it correct? ---- 113
- **Diagnosis, Signs & Symptoms** ---- 113
20. What are the sounds that we hear while measuring BP with the stethoscope? ---- 113
21. Can we measure BP without Stethoscope? ---- 113
22. Can we measure our own BP by using stethoscope and BP machine? ---- 114
23. What are the kinds of BP apparatus available in the market? Which one is better? ---- 114
24. What happens during High BP? ---- 114
25. What are the causes of high BP? ---- 114
26. What are the symptoms of high BP? ---- 115
27. How to diagnose high BP? ---- 115
28. What is primary HT? ---- 115
29. What is secondary HT? ---- 115
30. What is white coat hypertension? ---- 115
31. What are the tests to be done in high BP? ---- 115
32. What is ambulatory BP measurement? ---- 116
33. Which BP machine is better - Mercury or Diet type? ---- 116
34. Can we depend on electronic BP machines? ---- 116
35. How often can BP be measured? ---- 116
36. What should be the aim of treatment of HT? ---- 117

37. How to treat HT? ---- 117
38. What role does medicine play in HT? ---- 117
39. Which medicines can be used in HT? ---- 117
40. What are diuretics? Give some examples. ---- 117
41. What are Beta blockers? Give some examples. ---- 118
42. What are Alpha blockers? Give some examples. ---- 118
43. What are calcium channel blockers? Give some examples. ---- 118
44. What are ACE inhibitors? Give some examples. ---- 118
45. What are Angiotensin-II receptor blockers? Give some examples. ---- 119
46. What are Central acting agent drugs? Give some examples. ---- 119
47. What are Vasodilators? Give some examples. ---- 119
48. How to tackle HT in emergency? ---- 119
49. How long should the medication for lowering the BP continue? ---- 119
50. Do HT drugs have side effects? ---- 120
51. What are the side effects of Diuretics? ---- 120
52. What are the side effects of Beta Blockers? ---- 120
53. What are the side effects of ACE Inhibitors? ---- 120
54. What are the side effects of Angiotensin II receptor blockers? ---- 120
55. What are the side effects of Alpha Blockers? ---- 120
56. What are the side effects of central acting agents? ---- 120
57. What are the side effects of Vasodilators? ---- 121
58. Is it safe to take HT drugs in a long term? ---- 121
59. Can these drugs be combined together? ---- 121
60. Can the medicines for BP be stopped at any time in one's life? ---- 121
61. Do we need to reduce these medicines once the BP comes down to 120/80 mmHg or below? ---- 121
62. What to do if the BP is 120/80 mmHg? ---- 121
63. What to do if the BP goes below 120/80 mmHg? ---- 122

- **Diet & Hypertension**

64. Can a HT patient use salt in food preparation? ---- 122
65. What is salt sensitive HT? ---- 122
66. What is salt insensitive HT? ---- 122
67. How does high fiber diet help to reduce the HT? ---- 123
68. Can HT patient take tea or coffee more than 1-2 times in a day? ---- 123
69. Can a high cholesterol diet increase the BP? ---- 123
70. What do you mean by DASH diet? ---- 123
71. What are basic advices by DASH diet? ---- 123
72. What is a combination diet? ---- 124
73. Why combination diet is useful for HT patient? ---- 124
74. Why combination diet is better in HT patient? ---- 124
75. What are the sources of Calcium? ---- 124
76. What are the sources of magnesium ? ---- 125
77. What are the sources of potassium? ---- 126
78. What are Antioxidants? ---- 126
79. What are the sources of Antioxidants? ---- 126
80. Do Antioxidants also help in reducing HT?. ---- 126

- **Obesity & High BP**

81. How is obesity responsible for HT? ---- 127
82. How to rule out the obesity in a person? ---- 127
83. What is BMI? ---- 127
84. How to reduce the obesity? ---- 128
85. How can you differentiate over weight & obesity? ---- 128
86. In addition to high blood pressure, which other diseases do obesity lead to? ---- 128
87. Does BMI differ in male & female? ---- 128

- **Coronary Artery Disease & Hypertension**

88. What is CAD? ---- 128
89. What is MI? ---- 129
90. How HT is responsible for CAD or MI? ---- 129
91. Is HT only responsible for development of coronary heart disease? ---- 129
92. How much BP is safe for CAD patients? ---- 130

93. How to control the BP for CAD patient? ---- 130

- **Hypertension & Stroke/CVA**

94. How does HT lead to stroke/CVA? ---- 130
95. What is CVA? ---- 130
96. What is paralysis (Stroke)? ---- 131
97. How to reduce the BP? ---- 131
98. What is the treatment of CVA? ---- 131
99. What are the types of paralysis? ---- 131
100. What is hemiplegia? ---- 131
101. What is paraplegia? ---- 132
102. What is hemiparesis? ---- 132
103. What are the precautions to prevent CVA? ---- 132
104. What is TIA? ---- 132

- **Hypertension in Young**

105. Why hypertension occurs in young? ---- 133
106. Causes of HT in young people? ---- 133
107. How can BP problem be solved in young people? ---- 133
108. What should be the ideal BP in young? ---- 133
109. What are the complications of HT in Young? ---- 134

- **Exercise & High BP**

110. Does exercise reduce the BP? ---- 134
111. What are the exercises for reducing the BP? ---- 134
112. How much exercise should one do? ---- 134
113. Does yoga reduce the BP? ---- 134
114. Does pranayama reduce BP? ---- 135

- **Causes of Hypertension (HT)**

115. What are the causes of HT? ---- 135
116. Does stress lead to HT? ---- 135
117. Does Alcohol lead to HT? ---- 135
118. Does smoking cause HT? ---- 136
119. Do irregular exercises causes HT? ---- 136
120. Can taking improper food cause HT? ---- 136
121. Is heredity also a cause of HT? ---- 136

- **Stress & Hypertension (HT)**

122. What are the causes of stress in our daily life? ---- 136

123. How does stress cause HT? ---- 137
124. What happens when we are in stress? ---- 137
125. How can stress be reduced? ---- 137
126. How do we come to know that BP is due to stress? ---- 138
127. How does yoga help in HT? ---- 138
128. How does meditation help to reduce Stress? ---- 138
129. What is Kayotsarg? ---- 139
130. How can stress be managed? ---- 139
131. How much stress do I have? ---- 139
132. What is subconscious stress? ---- 140
133. How to know if I am under stress? ---- 140
134. How much time should I spend on meditation, kayotsarg? ---- 140
135. Can stress management cure HT? ---- 140
136. Why do people fight? ---- 140
137. How to manage financial stress? ---- 141
138. Does Satsang help to reduce stress? ---- 141
139. How to control Ego? ---- 141
140. How to speak so that it does not cause stress? ---- 142
141. Why does blood pressure rise when going for an interview or an exam? ---- 142

- **Miscellaneous**

142. What is the BP in lungs? ---- 142
143. What is Pulmonary HT? ---- 142
144. What are the symptoms of Pulmonary HT? ---- 143
145. What are the causes of Pulmonary HT? ---- 143
146. What is the treatment of Pulmonary HT? ---- 143
147. Can BP differ if measured in both arms? ---- 143
148. Can BP be measured in the legs? ---- 144
149. Does BP differ in the upper arms and legs? ---- 144
150. If a person is grossly obese then how to measure BP? ---- 144
151. What is the normal BP in children? ---- 144
152. Does obesity lead to HT? ---- 144

- **Heart & Its functions**

153. What are the functions of the heart? ---- 144

154. How is heart responsible in increasing the BP? ---- 145
155. How does High BP affect the heart? ---- 145
• **Low BP**
156. What is low BP or hypotension? ---- 145
157. How can we identify low BP? ---- 146
158. What are the causes of low BP? ---- 146
159. What is an ideal BP? ---- 146
160. How can low BP be treated? ---- 146
161. What to do if the BP falls suddenly? ---- 146
• **Renal Hypertension (HT)**
162. What is Renal HT or renal vascular HT? ---- 147
163. What are the causes of Renal HT? ---- 147
164. What are the symptoms of Renal HT? ---- 147
165. How does HT affect kidneys? ---- 148
166. What diet should patient take in renal HT? ---- 148
167. At what age does renal HT mostly occur? ---- 148
168. Who can suffer from Renal HT? ---- 148
169. Does obesity affect Renal HT? ---- 148
170. What is the treatment for Renal HT? ---- 148
• **Complications of Hypertension (HT)**
171. What are the complications of HT? ---- 149
172. How does HT affect the Heart? ---- 149
173. How does HT affect the brain? ---- 150
174. How does HT affect the eyes? ---- 150
175. Why do Patients with HT get a cardiac arrest? ---- 150
176. Why is it necessary to control the BP before a Surgery? --- 150
• **Women & Hypertension (HT)**
177. What is the normal BP for women? ---- 151
178. Why does high Blood Pressure occur in women? ---- 151
179. What is Pre delivery HT? ---- 151
180. What is Post delivery HT? ---- 151
181. Should we use medicine to control Pre delivery HT? ---- 152
182. What happens to this kind of HT after delivery? ---- 152
183. Does diet control give some relief in post delivery HT? --- 152
184. Do oral contraceptive pills increase the BP? ---- 152

185. Does menopause affect HT in women? ---- 152

- **Alternative Therapies & Hypertension (HT) control**

186. What is the alternative treatment for HT? ---- 153
187. Does yoga help to control HT? ---- 153
188. Does regular exercise control HT? ---- 153
189. Does regular walking help to control HT? ---- 154
190. Does meditation help to control HT? ---- 154
191. Does kayotsarg help to control HT? ---- 154

- **DM & HT**

192. What is Diabetes? ---- 154
193. What are the symptoms of diabetes? ---- 155
194. What is the normal Blood Sugar level? ---- 155
195. How does Diabetes Mellitus lead to HT? ---- 155
196. Why do Diabetes Mellitus patients usually become hypertensive? ---- 156
197. What diet should be given to a patient with Diabetes Mellitus and High BP? ---- 156
198. Can exercise help to reduce the HT in the diabetic patients? ---- 156
199. Can Yoga help to reduce HT in diabetic patients? ---- 156
200. How is HT controlled in a diabetic patients? ---- 156
201. What are the medicines to be used in patients with High BP and High Blood Sugar? ---- 157

Chapter-1

Understanding Blood Pressure & Hypertension

1. WORKING OF THE CARDIOVASCULAR SYSTEM

(a) Cardiovascular System

> **1. Working of the Cardiovascular System.**
> **2. Risk factors for High BP.**
> **3. Common knowledge about High BP.**
> **4. Types of High Blood Pressure.**

Cardiovascular system includes heart, blood vessels which circulate blood to different parts of your body. Heart is divided into four chambers and with each beat of your heart a constant quantity of blood is released from heart's fourth chamber (left ventricle) which is also known as pumping chamber of the heart. The blood is thrown into the blood vessels that spread throughout your body. The main function of the blood is to carry food to different parts of body for the proper functioning of systems in your body. Aorta, largest artery, is connected to the left ventricle and serves as the main channel for blood leaving your heart. The aorta further divides into smaller arteries, which in turn divide into even smaller arteries known as arterioles.

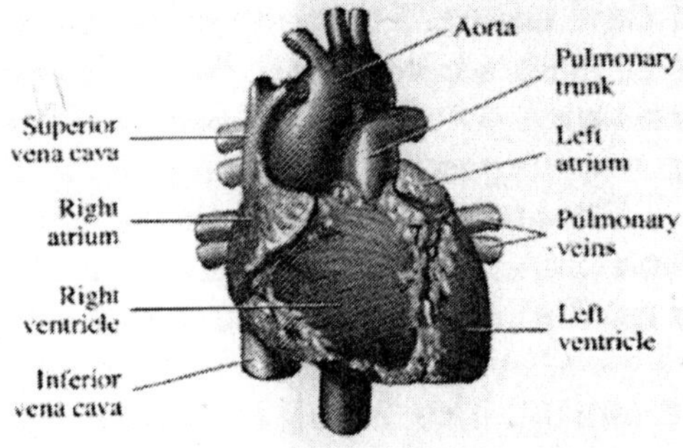

In our body there are very small tubes we can't see with

our naked eyes known as capillaries. These vessels can be seen with microscope and the main function of these tubes is the exchange of tiny food particles and oxygen. Oxygen and food is delivered to every cell of the body and waste products are collected back by these capillaries.

The blood from the different parts of the body is collected through other type of vessels known as veins and is sent back to the heart. From heart blood is routed to lungs, where it releases carbon dioxide and picks up oxygen. The process is known as gaseous exchange. This freshly oxygenated blood is sent back to the heart, ready to begin another journey.

(b) What is High Blood pressure or Hypertension?

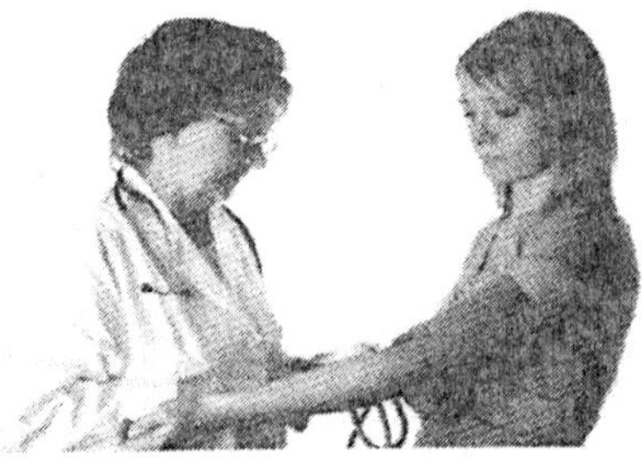

Hypertension or High blood pressure is the increment of the pressure exerted by the flowing blood on the walls of the tubes(arteries) that carry the blood from the heart to every part of the body.

To understand blood pressure and the effects of it on different organs one must know the regulation of blood pressure in the body. The following information will make it easy for you to understand how high blood pressure develops and why it can be so dangerous.

(c) Need for Blood Pressure:

Any liquid flows from high pressure zone to low pressure zone. As far as the flow of blood in our body is concerned an initial pressure head has to be created. When the left ventricle of the heart pumps some blood into the already filled arterial system – a high pressure in created . This pushes blood towards the low pressure zone. So, the blood flows a little. But immediately the ventricle contracts again. So, another bout of flow occurs. The contraction goes indefinitely this way and thus establishes a continuous flow of blood throughout the body. ***Blood pressure is the amount of pressure exerted by blood to facilitate blood in reaching to the different parts of the body.***

The pressure at the main tubes of the body when the heart (Left Ventricle) contracts is equivalent to 120 millimeter of Mercury(written as mmHg) and is called the systolic pressure. As this pressure pushes the blood away from the heart to the small arteries this pressure falls to 80 mmHg. This is called Diastolic pressure. By that time the left ventricle pumps again more blood into the system creating one more wave of higher Blood pressure. So the pressure keeps on fluctuating between 120 and 80 mmHg with every contraction and relaxation of the heart.This can be felt if you feel your pulse in the wrist. It is this pressure that keeps on moving the blood throughout our body. The work of the flowing blood is to deliver the food and oxygen to the cells of the body and come back again to the heart through tubes known as Veins to be pushed again.

All-together our arteries and veins have about 5 liters of blood at a time and with every contraction the left ventricle pushes some 70 ml of blood with a higher pressure of 120 mmHg. The next moment it again receives another 70 ml to be pushed again. This goes on and on. Without this blood pressure the flow of blood would not have happened and we would have been dead.

(d) The Organs that control Blood Pressure:

The Five major organs that help to control your blood pressure are heart, kidney, arteries, nervous system and hormones.

Heart:

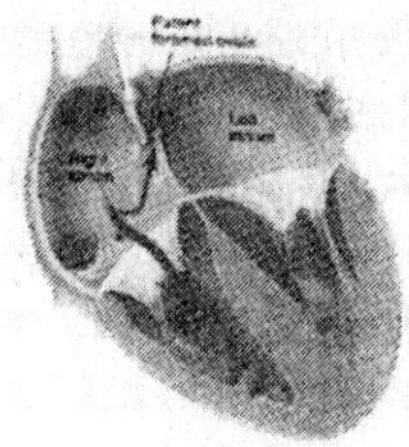

Heart is a muscular organ. When these muscles contract, a force is created sufficient to eject the blood into the main artery (aorta). The harder your heart muscle has to work to release the blood, the greater the force is exerted on the arteries.

Arteries:

Arteries are blood carrying tubes from the heart to the parts of the body. Smaller arteries are called Arteriols and capillaries. These arteries are lined by smooth muscles that allow them to contract and expand as blood passes. The more elastic your arteries are, the less resistant they are to the flow of blood and less force that is exerted on their walls. When arteries loose their elasticity or become narrowed, resistance to blood flow increases and additional force is needed to push blood through the vessels. These arteries are also supplied by the nerves of the Sympathetic Nervous System. These nerves– when stimulated lead to constriction of the arteries leading to Higher Blood pressure.

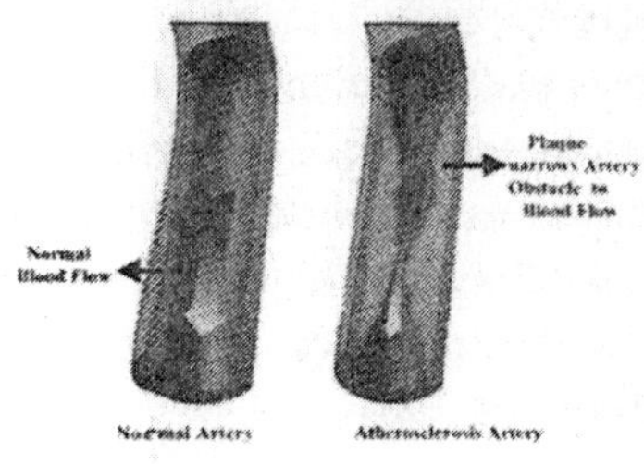

Kidneys:

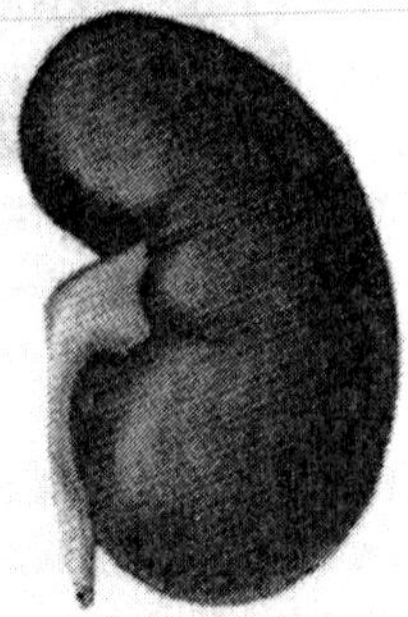

One of the main functions of kidneys is to maintain the volume of water at normal level and regulate the amount of sodium in the body. Water is dependent on sodium. If there is retention of sodium, it retains more water in the body. This extra fluid can overload your blood vessels and increase blood pressure. The kidneys also release some chemicals called Angiotensinogen which also has a major role to play in the control of Blood pressure. Some enzymes called ACE (Angiotensinogen Converting enzyme) help is increasing the action of these released chemicals released from the kidneys.

Nervous system:

The Nervous system which is controlled by the brain and the nerves which encircle the spinal cord (called Sympathetic Nervous system) play a major role in control of our Blood pressure. The nervous system releases neurotransmitters which can stimulate a organ called Hypothalamus which control the emotional brain. Whenever the hypothalamus is excited there is release of many hormones into the blood stream which lead to contraction of the arteries leading to high BP. The nerves also control the proteins (receptors) called alpha and beta receptors which stimulate the heart –leading to increased contraction and increases rate of the heart. This also leads to high BP.

All our stress and tensions are mediated through the brain and nervous system. So, directly or indirectly our stress or psychological pressure is translated to High BP through the nervous system.

Hormones:

Our hormones also control our BP through their action on the heart, on the arteries and nerves. The main among them is adrenaline (called Epinephrine) – which is called the stress hormone. Whenever they are secreted they lead to increased heart rate, increased contraction of the heart and squeezing of the arteries. When to cut down the stress the immediate effect is lowering of the BP. Cortisol, ACTH, Aldosterone, Thyroxine – are some of the hormones which play an important role in controlling of BP. Many new hormones and neuro hormones have been discovered by the medical science in recent days which have various effects on BP.

2. CAUSES OR RISK FACTORS FOR HIGH BLOOD PRESSURE

High BP is not caused by a single reason, but many factors together lead to increment of blood pressure. These causes are known as Risk factors for High BP. These risk factors can be divided into two major groups – *Modifiable* and *Non Modifiable*. Non modifiable causes can not be changed. But the modifiable causes are much more common and can be changed – by our own efforts.

(a) Non-modifiable risk factors :

These are the risk factors you can't change. It means that there is no medicine to keep them in control. These risk factors are:

i) **Age :** With age BP rises in both male and female.

ii) **Genetic Factors:** The importance of genetic factors in increasing BP has been confirmed. Studies have shown that the children of normotensive parents (BP within normal limits) have 3 per cent possibility of developing high BP, whereas this possibility is 45 per cent in children of two high BP parents.

(b) Modifiable risk factors :

These are the risk factors you can change. The factors which come in this category are:

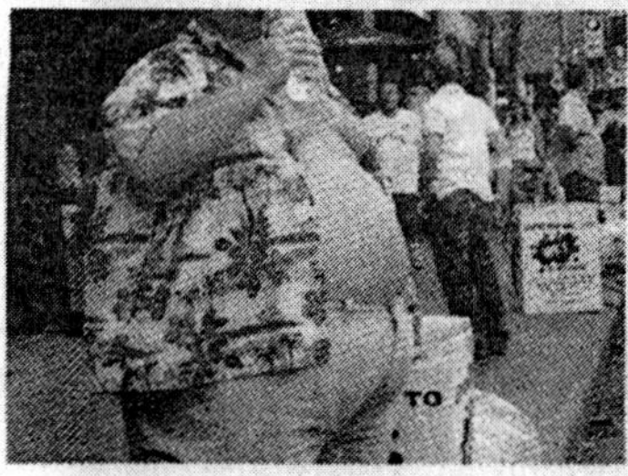

i.) Obesity : Obesity is one of the proven risk factors for high BP. With the increase in weight the risk for developing high BP increases. Research studies have shown that when people lose their weight their BP decreases.

ii.) Fats: Increased fat intake (both Cholesterol and Triglycerides) can raise blood pressure. Increased blood level of both Cholesterol and Triglycerides also lead to atherosclerosis and this also tends to increase the blood pressure.

iii.) Alcohol : High alcohol intake is associated with an increased risk of high BP. Recent studies have shown that high systolic BP is more dangerous than high diastolic BP. It appears that alcohol raises systolic pressure more than diastolic.

iv) Physical inactivity : It increases BP indirectly by increasing body weight and other unknown methods.

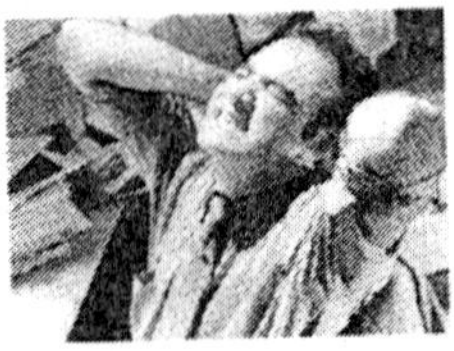

v) Psychological stress : In persons with stress there is over reactivity of the sympathetic nervous system. Due to this over reactivity more adrenalin is released in the blood and there is rise in BP.

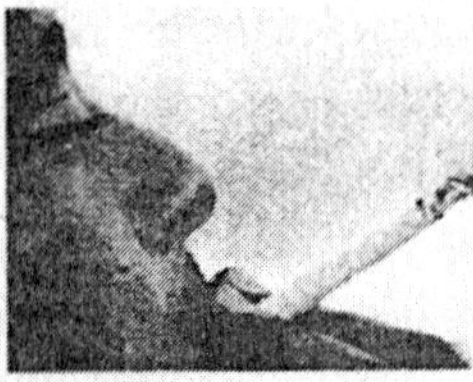

vi) Salt intake : Evidences show that high salt intake increases BP proportionally. For instance, the higher incidence of high BP is found in Japan where salt intake is more.

vii) Smoking: Smoking and tobacco intake has also been associated with high Blood Pressure.

vii) Other factors : Other factors which can raise BP are oral contraceptives, noise, vibration, temperature.

(C) Does Tension or Stress lead to Hypertension?

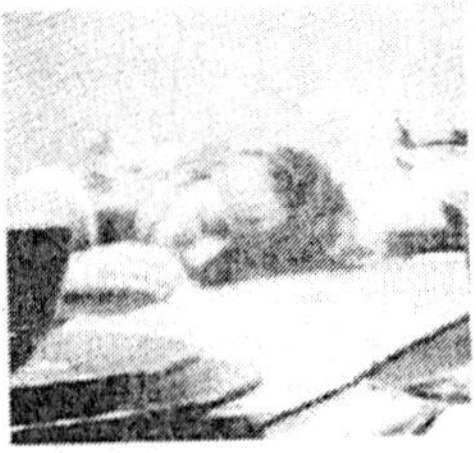

Does everyone at work have a say in how your job is done-except you? Does getting stuck in traffic makes you boil over, along with your radiator? Do you regularly get hot under the collar over things that other people just shrug off? If so, you're a candidate for one of the latest medical discoveries: stress-induced hypertension.

The Stress Reaction

Whenever you are under stress, your body starts a reaction called *Stress reaction*. It shoots your blood up with adrenaline, which raises your blood pressure, blood sugar and heart rate. It even increases your muscle tone. Blood pressure drops slowly, until the next aggravation comes along. Too much of this and the body gives up and boosts its baseline blood pressure to a permanently higher levels.

Stress and High Blood Pressure

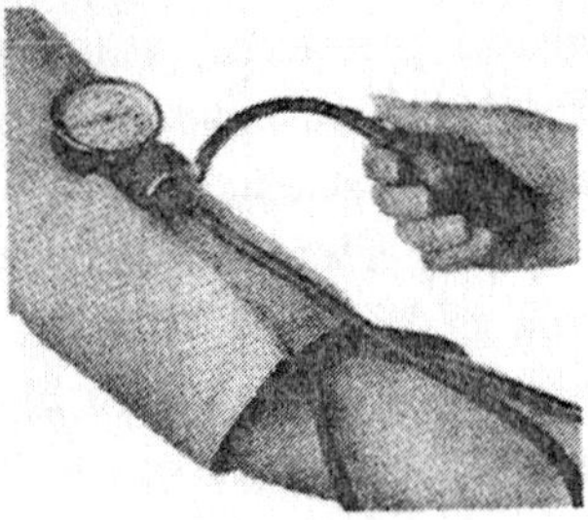

People who experience chronic stress are more likely to have chronically high blood pressure. How do you know if you suffer from chronic stress? It is simple: if you feel stressed out, you are. In fact, people vary widely in their reaction to stress. That's why, those who get upset easily are more likely to have stress-induced hypertension. It is now assumed that stress in life contributes to 50% of cause of high BP.

The Power of Adrenaline

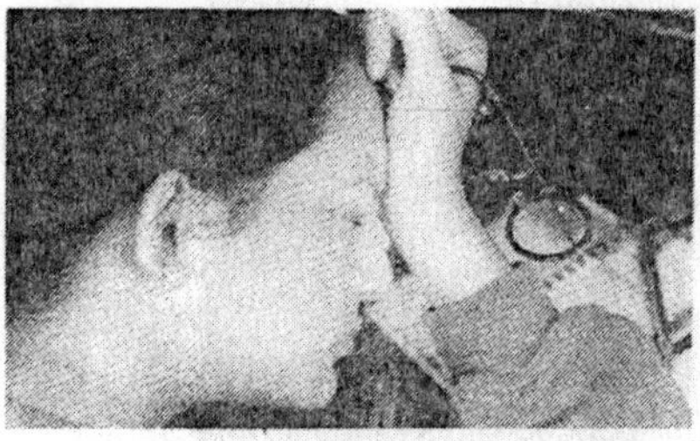

It has happened to everyone. It begins when you are startled, frightened or angry. Your heart pounds, your breath is shallow and you sweat profusely. Your intestines shut down. You feel tense, apprehensive and ready to respond to danger. The substance responsible for all these changes is *adrenaline,* a hormone, which your body secretes to give you the strength and alertness to fight off or escape danger. It's the classic **"fight or flight"** response and it was ideal when most of the dangers humans face were physical. By fighting or running away, people both resolve their problem and work off the tension that adrenaline produces.

Adrenaline also causes jitters when you are under stress, whether that stress directly threatens your safety or not. These stressful events could be being stuck in traffic, having a deadline to meet or conflict with family members. Even positive stresses, like a promotion or getting married, can affect you. Unfortunately, you can't respond to most stresses by running away or fighting them.

What can be done about stress?

A feeling of helplessness is one of the most common stressors in our society. But you don't have to be a helpless victim of stress induced hypertension. Stress management programs that exist can help you learn the fine art of relaxation. Techniques like deep breathing, progressive muscle relaxation & regular exercise can also help you let off your steam safely.

Get your blood pressure checked. If it's high, or if you feel too much under stress, ask your doctor where you can get into a stress-reduction program. Or maybe your workplace has a program. Start right now by taking a deep breath.

3. Common knowledge about High Blood Pressure

(a) What is Normal BP or High Blood Pressure?

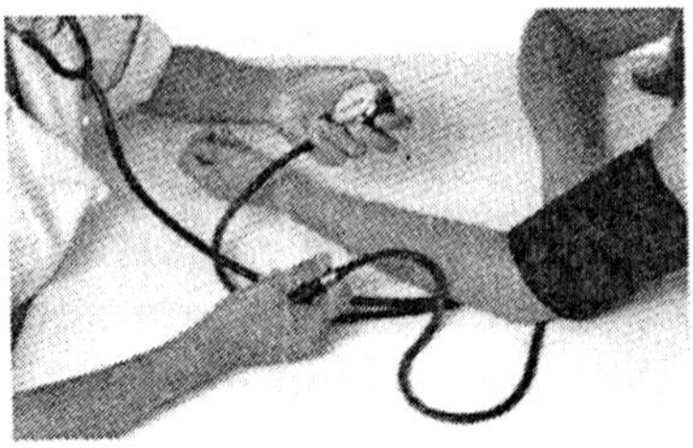

Normal BP: It is the amount of pressure exerted by blood on the walls of blood carrying vessels, enough to facilitate blood to reach to the different parts of the body. BP should be always less than 120/80 mmHg.

According to the data gathered from the Framingham Heart Study, 50 percent of people who have a first heart attack and two thirds of those who have a first stroke have blood pressures higher than 160/95 mm of Hg.

The incidence of hypertension among people in lower socio-economic groups is under estimated because of the inadequate access to medical care.

If left untreated, high blood pressure continues to rise gradually over the years, causing the heart to overwork itself to the point where serious damage can occur. Untreated hypertension also places other systems and organs (e.g., the kidneys) at greater risks of damage leading to dysfunction or failure of organ.

The most authentic agency to classify high BP in the whole of the world is Joint National Committee (JNC) of USA. In 1997 the sixth report of the JNC classified Hypertension in the following Categories.

Stage	Systolic Pressure (mm of Hg)	Diastolic Pressure
Best*	Under 120	Under 80
Normal	Under 130	Under 85
High Normal	130-139	85-89
Stage I	140-159	90-99
Stage II	160-179	100-109
Stage III	180-209	110-119
Stage IV	210 or above	120 or above

** Note: Optimal levels are with respect to heart disease risk. Not usually but low readings of BP can also negatively affect heart health and should be reported to a physician.*

Hypertension has often been called the **"silent killer"**, because mild to moderate levels usually go unnoticed by patients until serious damage has already been done. To clarify the risk factors, high blood pressure measurements for adults have been ranked according to risk categories of increasing severity, ranging from "normal" to "stage 4." An important exception, to the information listed above is noted among patients with diabetes and/or kidney disease. These patients require treatment, if their blood pressure rises above 130/80 mm of Hg.

(b) How is High Blood Pressure diagnosed?

While diagnosing hypertension, a physician considers the full medical history of a patient. For example, the physician will ask whether high blood pressure runs in the family and what the patient's dietary habits are (e.g., salt intake). The physician will also give the patient a complete physical examination, which will include checking the patient's blood pressure in both arms, while standing and lying down. In some cases, the physician may even ask the patient to take his or her own blood pressure at home and bring in a daily log of blood pressure measurements.

This strategy will help to establish the patient's normal blood pressure pattern and to rule out White Coat Hypertension (high blood pressure only while in a physician's office).

Once a diagnosis has been made and serious problems (like kidney disease) have been ruled out, then the treatment can begin. However, a very high blood pressure may require additional testing to rule out an unusual cause. For example, *a Renal Doppler Sonogram* or scan may be ordered to evaluate for high blood pressure due to disease of the blood vessels of the kidneys (renovascular hypertension). Also, a 24-hour urine test may be needed to rule out an endocrine disorder, such as Cushing Disease or Pheochromocytosis.

Hypertension may occur in either adults or children. Some people may also be diagnosed with the opposite condition: low blood pressure (hypotension). Although some hypertensives do not need to take medication, as long as they can control their risk factors (e.g., weight). Most cases generally require long-term treatment with medications.

(c) What are the symptoms of High Blood Pressure?

The majority of people with mild to moderate hypertension cannot tell when their blood pressure is too high. In fact, about one-third of hypertensive people are not aware of their condition. Patients may experience chest pain (angina), shortness of breath or other symptoms related to heart disease. If you have some of the difficulties listed below you should check your BP immediately.

Symptoms

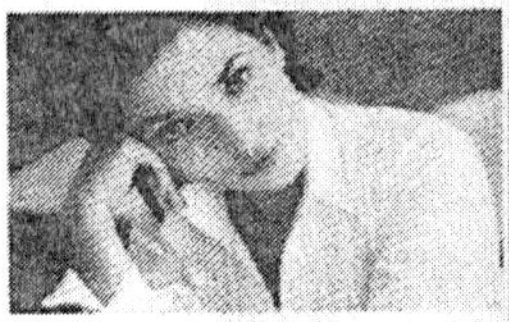

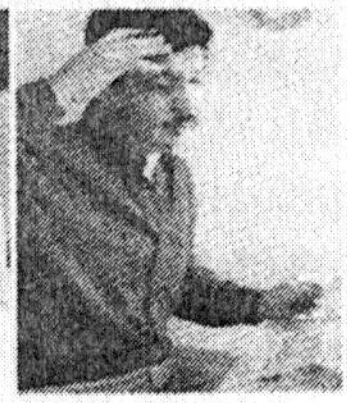

1. Fatigue
2. Confusion
3. Nausea or upset stomach
4. Vision changes or problems
5. Excessive sweating
6. Paleness or redness of skin
7. Nose bleeding
8. Anxiety or nervousness
9. Palpitations (strong, fast or obviously irregular heartbeat)
10. Ringing or buzzing in ears
11. Impotence
12. Headache
13. Dizziness

If you discover one day that you have High BP you should undergo the following tests also to know the reason or know the extent of damage by the blood pressure so far.

Tests

1. **Urine Analyser** and various blood tests (e.g., electrolytes and waste products test to rule out kidney disease, serum lipid profile).
2. **Electrocardiogram (ECG)**, which measures the heart's electrical activity. By analyzing the ECG results, a physician can check for heart-related problems that could be associated with high blood pressure (e.g., left ventricular hypertrophy).

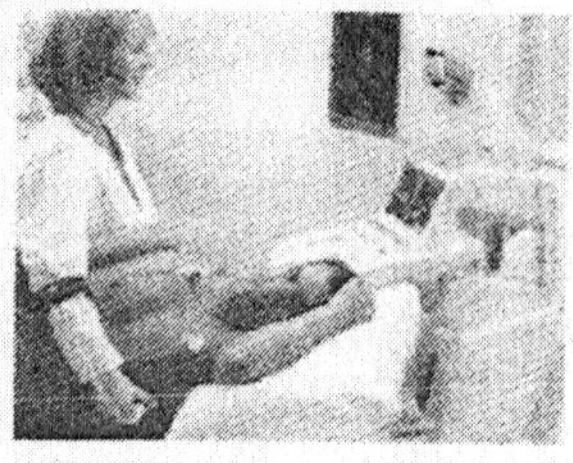

3. **Echocardiogram**, which uses sound waves to visualize the structures and functions of the heart. This test is also used to check for heart-related problems such as left ventricular hypertrophy.
4. **Chest x-ray** to rule out an enlarged heart.

TYPES OF HYPERTENSION

There are different types of hypertensions, which are as follows: primary, secondary, renovascular, labile, malignant and resistant. Until the year 2000, these different types were generally diagnosed by paying attention to people's diastolic blood pressure (the lower number of a blood pressure reading). In other words, someone with "high blood pressure" actually had diastolic hypertension. However, the National Heart Lung and Blood Institute of USA recommended that healthcare professionals should evaluate not only systolic blood pressure, but also their diastolic blood pressure while making a diagnosis of hypertension. Nowadays, syotolic BP is considered more important than diastolic blood pressure.

Most people with high blood pressure are diagnosed with primary hypertension, which means that researchers only understand the risk factors for the condition but not the root cause. However, these people show substantial improvement with stress management techniques.

Primary (Essential) Hypertension

- Though the main causes of High Blood Pressure is excessive stress, excess weight, and lack of exercise and so on, our medical science describes 90-95% of High Blood Pressure cases as Primary, or Essential Hypertension. The rest 5-10% are called Secondary Hypertension – where the cause is very much clear (like Kidney disease, drug induced High BP). The following are factors that are associated with essential hypertension and may increase the risk of developing the condition:

- Stress
- Family history of hypertension
- Obesity.
- Lack of regular exercise
- Smoking
- Advanced age.
- High caffeine intake
- Diet high in fats and oils
- High cholesterol levels
- Inherited problems in the body's angiotensin-renin system, which influences all factors related to controlling blood pressure: blood vessel contraction, heart cell development, sodium and water balance and the "salt genes" which play an important role in the relationship between salt and hypertension.

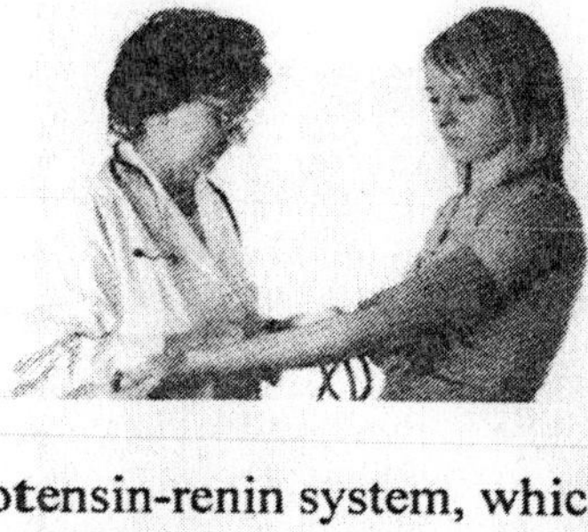

Inherited problems in the body's sympathetic nervous system, include those which control heart rate, blood pressure and the width of blood vessels.

What is Secondary hypertension?

Secondary hypertension is a condition in which the cause of the high blood pressure is known (e.g., sleep, apnea or some form of kidney or endocrine diseases). The high blood pressure is secondary to another disease or disorder and the hypertension usually disappears once the underlying condition is controlled or cured. These underlying conditions include the following:

- Sleep
- Kidney or endocrine disease
- Cirrhosis of the liver
- Cushing disease (in which the body produces excess steroids)
- Pheochromocytoma (adrenaline-producing tumor)
- Coarctation of the aorta (a condition in which the aorta is pinched, constricted or narrowed at some point along its length, often resulting in high blood pressure in the arms and low blood pressure in the legs).

Some more Factors that could cause secondary hypertension

1. **Pregnancy (pregnancy-induced hypertension)**: Pregnancy can worsen the hypertension of women who already have it, or cause hypertension in women with no history of it. After the delivery, hypertension tends to resolve in women with no prior history of it. However, women who develop hypertension during pregnancy are likely to develop it again later in life.

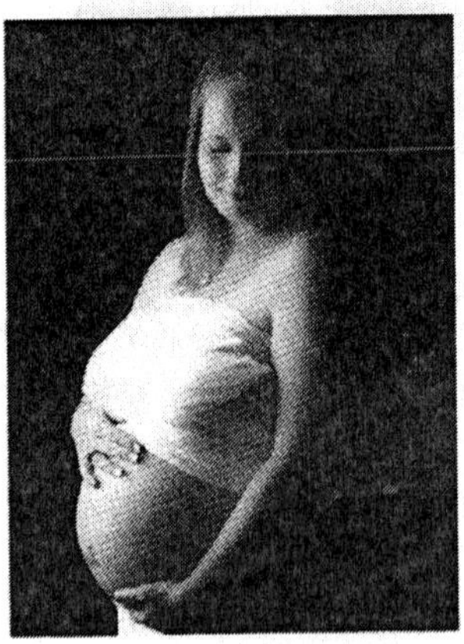

2. **Certain medications**: Prescribed medications that can cause temporarily high blood pressure include certain Non Steroidal Anti-Inflammatory drugs (NSAIDs) and estrogen (in either oral contraceptives or hormone replacement therapy). Over the counter (OTC) medications that can cause

the same effect include NSAIDS (e.g., ibuprofen or naproxen), cold, cough and sinus medications and many eye drops.

3. **Cocaine use :** Not only can cocaine cause blood pressure to rise sharply, but it can also cause heart attack and stroke in healthy people of any age.

4. **Alcohol** : Long-term overuse of alcohol, caffeine or real licorice, which contain a steroid-like substance can cause HT.

Some more types of Hypertension

Renovascular hypertension is one of the most common forms of secondary hypertension and is caused due to decreased blood flow to the kidneys. Usually, this blood flow gets restricted when the arteries to the kidneys become narrow(renal artery stenosis). Renal blood vessels narrow down due to one of the two following conditions — *atherosclerosis or fibromuscular dysplasia*. Atherosclerosis is a disease in which arteries become hardened and narrowed, as a result of plaque that has build up along the inside of the artery walls. Fibromuscular dysplasia is a condition in which cells from the artery walls overgrow, causing the arteries to narrow down.

Isolated Systolic Hypertension

Isolated systolic hypertension (ISH) is when only systolic blood pressure (the larger number of a blood pressure reading) is elevated. ISH occurs mainly in older people because systolic pressure increases with age while diastolic pressure usually declines after the age of 55. ISH patients have a rise in systolic pressure (above 140) but diastolic pressure remains normal. ISH is a common cause of stroke.

Labile or Transient Hypertension

Labile or transient, hypertension is a temporary rise in blood pressure during stressful situations. Blood pressure then returns to normal.

Many young people who have labile hypertension for several years and go on to develop primary hypertension, especially if they have a family history of hypertension. However, even labile hypertension may result in complications such as heart disease, kidney disease and stroke, if left untreated. It is often treated successfully with beta blockers or other medications and stress management.

Resistant Hypertension

Resistant hypertension is high blood pressure that does not respond to typical treatments and therapies. Because of this, it is difficult to control and often requires lifestyle changes and two or three different medications in order to properly treat this condition. People with resistant hypertension, are urged to work closely with the physician who manages their condition and are advised to very carefully follow all of the physician's orders regarding diet, exercise and medications.

Malignant (Accelerated) Hypertension

Malignant or accelerated hypertension occurs in less than one percent of hypertensive patients. It is defined as a sudden rise in diastolic blood pressure to over 125. This very high diastolic blood pressure can be associated with damage to the brain, heart, eyes and kidneys. The condition is considered life threatening and immediate medical attention is extremely important. Treatment generally, requires intensive care hospitalization with potent medications delivered through an intravenous (I.V.) line to take effect as quickly as possible. Symptoms include loss of vision, nausea, drowsiness, confusion and headache.

White Coat Hypertension

Some people - knowingly or unknowingly - become anxious, when they have their blood pressure measured in hospital setup. These people may have normal blood pressure at other times, but when it is measured in a medical setting, it is always high. This condition is called "white-coat hypertension" and is fairly common.

If your doctor suspects your high blood pressure is white-coat hypertension, then you may need to measure your blood pressure at home and keep a note of your reading. Or your doctor may recommend that you wear a portable device (ambulatory monitor) that measures your blood pressure periodically throughout the day while you go about your regular activities. These two methods generally give a more realistic and accurate assessment of your blood pressure.

❑

Chapter-2

Blood Pressure Measurement

Blood pressure is generally measured by using an instrument called **Sphygmomanometer** medically. It also needs a stethoscope. This measurement takes only a few minutes and can be taught to anyone with a little training. These instruments can be bought by a patient who has High BP for about Rs.1000. Before you start measurement please go through the theory of BP measurement.

GENERAL TECHNIQUE

Blood pressure is measured by wrapping an arm cuff (attached to a sphygmomanometer) around the patient's arm and then using a stethoscope to listen to the brachial artery located at the inside elbow on the same arm. The cuff is then pumped full of air until circulation is very briefly cut off. Then some air will be slowly let out of the device, loosening the cuff's grip on the arm and releasing the blood to flow freely again. As the air is let out, the examiner watches the numbers coming down on a simple monitor (sphygmomanometer) and waits until he or she hears the first heart beat. The number at which it is heard is the systolic pressure. The examiner remembers this as the numbers continue to come down on the monitor and notes the number at which he or she hears the last heartbeat. The number at which that occurs is the diastolic pressure.

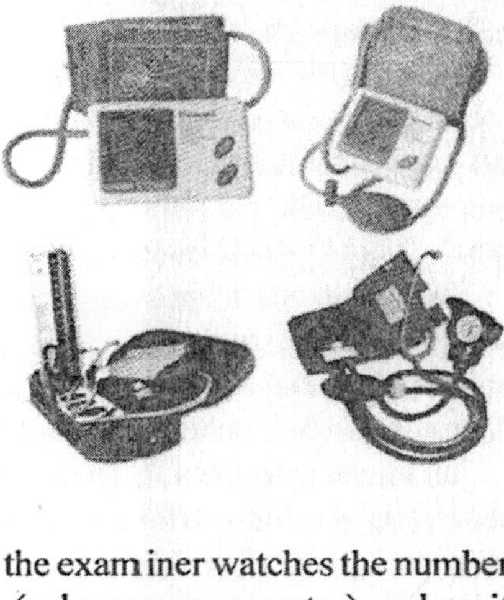

UNDERSTANDING THE TECHNIQUE OF MEASUREMENT OF BP

Blood flows into our hands through brachial artery which enters the arm after arising from the main supply line of the body called Aorta. This artery can be felt with our fingers just above the elbow joint. A branch of the same artery called Radial artery can also be felt flowing the blood at the wrist. When we want to measure the pressure of flowing blood in these tubes we squeeze the brachial artery by a cuff applied on the arm on the underlying arm bone (called Humerus). When the applied pressure exceeds the Blood pressure the flow of the blood to the arm is stopped. We have to usually feel the artery pulse disappear as the pressure is increased by the cuff.

Now the pressure of the cuff is gradually released and we put a stethoscope chest piece on the pulse area and hear the sound of flowing blood. As soon as the applied pressure falls just below the systolic pressure the blood flow of the brachial artery will start - and this flow being turbulent will lead to sounds which can be picked up by the stethoscope. This will be a ticking sound to begin with. At this time the pressure is noted in the pressure meter attached to the cuff. This is the Systolic pressure.

Now the pressure of the cuff is gradually lowered and the sound is monitored. As soon as we reach the diastolic pressure– the blood flow will have no obstruction and the flow will be streamlined which do not give any sound. So as soon as the sound disappears the pressure is noted . This is the Diastolic pressure.

When we start learning the measurement of Blood pressure we need more practice which make us conversant with the application of the cuff, slow and steady, release of pressure and listening of the sounds. After about 10-15 times of practice the person is almost trained.

To know how BP fluctuates throughout the day, BP monitoring is also available. Many clinicians now prefer to treat BP patients after a complete knowledge about the BP variations in the whole of the day.

TYPES OF BLOOD PRESSURE EQUIPMENTS:

1. Mercury Sphygmomanometer : This has a mercury column and is available in steel boxes. This has a tube, a cuff and a rubber bulb. This is the best and most dependable type of BP measuring equipment. Such machines are best for home use. You need to buy a stethoscope with this. This machine is not suitable for travel as it is heavy, bulky and has chances of breakage.

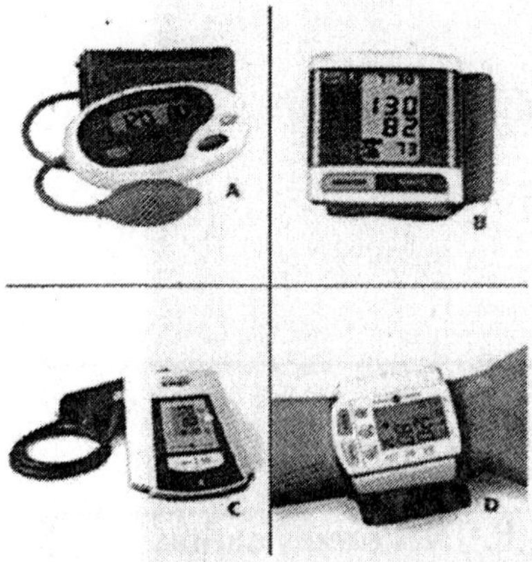

2. Dial Type Portable Sphygmomanometer: This has become more popular these days. Instead of Mercury column it has a pointer needle. If you buy it remember they must be of good quality. They have low weight, are small and can be carried to any place comfortably. You also need a stethoscope with it.

3. Electronic or Digital automatic BP machines: These do not need any expertise to measure also. The machine has a microphone which picks up the sounds in the brachial artery and give you a measurement. It also inflates and deflates the cuff automatically. These machines may not be accurate always – so before you buy – please cross check the readings with a doctor's measurement. If the readings are matching – you can buy. It usually costs Rs.2500.

DO'S AND DON'TS ABOUT BP MEASUREMENTS:

1. Blood pressure is best measured after at least five minutes of rest or quiet sitting.
2. Two readings three minutes apart are desirable, especially for those under stress.
3. The cuff should be at the level of the heart.
4. Blood pressure should be measured at least one hour after taking meals or tea or coffee intake.
5. The bladder inside the cuff should cover at 80% of the upper arm.
6. BP measurement should not be measured for at least 30 minutes after smoking.

❑

Chapter-3

Plan of Treatment of High Blood Pressure

1. Diet modification
2. Management of stress
3. Exercise & physical activity
4. Quit smoking
5. Abstinence from Alcohol
6. Yoga
7. Meditation
8. Weight reduction
9. Drugs (if required)

Control of high blood pressure can be successfully achieved by diet changes, weight reduction, stress management training, exercise promotion, behavioural changes and health education. These can be called Non Drug Therapy or Lifestyle Changes. But if still BP can not be controlled we should use medicines which are widely available.

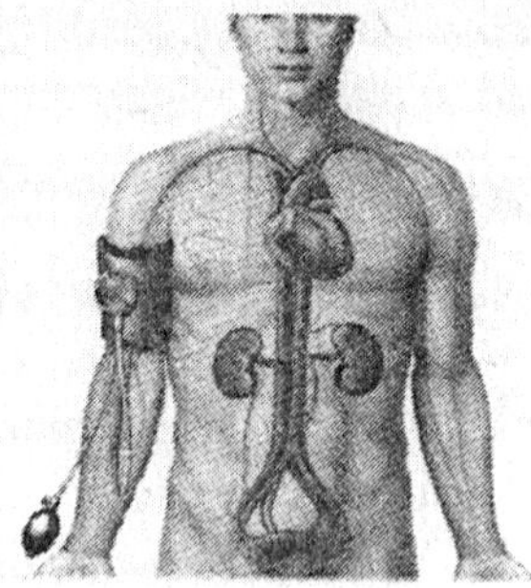

DIET FOR HIGH BP MANAGEMENT:

The diet changes for a high Blood pressure patient includes the following which is discussed in detail in the following chapters.

Gist for Diet Plan

a. Restriction of salts
b. Restriction of calories for those who are overweight
c. Restriction of fats
d. High fibre diet
e. Diet high in antioxidants

STRESS MANAGEMENT:

Management of stress is the most important way to control your Blood pressure. In fact 50% of Blood pressure patients can be controlled completely with stress management – if they can be implemented in their life. Stress management techniques include the following:

a. Training of the Rational Brain and Taming our Emotional mind.
b. Understanding stress and its effects on our life.
c. Identifying the role of our surroundings in production of stress and how to handle these external factors.
d. Understanding our attitude, desires, reactions, wants and the mindset. Modification of our mindset.
e. Avoiding the overloads of life.
f. Balancing the sectors of our life.
g. Release and management of stress.
h. Improving the way we speak.

EXERCISE

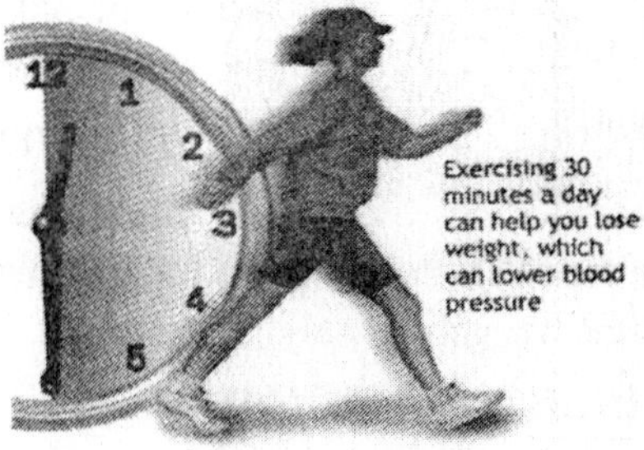
12
1
2
3
4
5
Exercising 30 minutes a day can help you lose weight, which can lower blood pressure

Exercise promotion leads to reduction or fall in body weight, blood lipids & blood pressure. Walking is the best kind of exercise for a hypertension patient. Other kinds of exercises like Yogic stretching, aerobics, cycling, swimming are good ways to reduce Blood pressure. These exercises only give effects if they are done regularly and for atleast 30 minutes per day.

CESSATION OF SMOKING

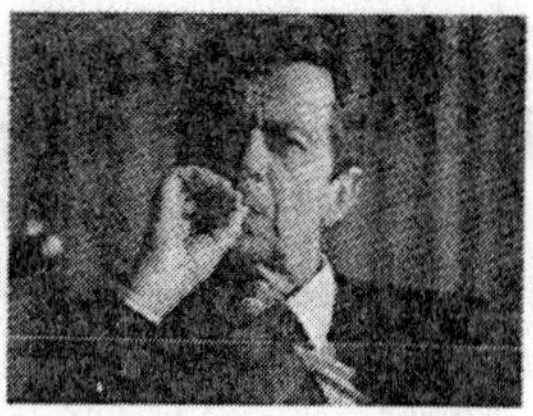

Different types of smoking - cigarette, cigar, bidi, hooka etc. contain nicotine. This nicotine gets accumulated in the intimal layer of vessels (inner most layer of arteries) due to which the inner surface which was smooth becomes rough and makes a good medicine for the accumulation of fats & this way helps in the formulation of blockages.

It also makes the vessels stiff so they lose their elasticity due to which vessel can burst and their can be bleeding mostly in nose and brain.

Smoking causes hypertension which may lead to angina and finally heart attack.

ALCOHOL

It has been observed that persons who consume alcohol regularly, invariably suffer from high blood pressure. One should avoid consumption of alcohol.

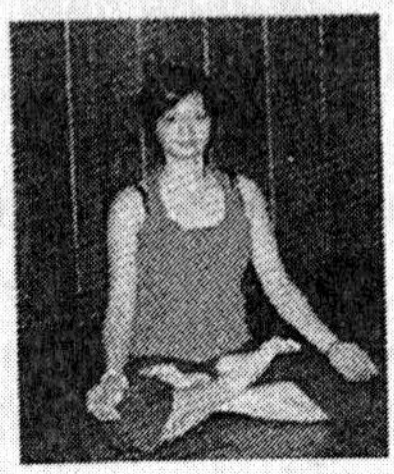

YOGA

It is advocated for mental relaxation as it helps in improving personal response to the environment. There are various asanas which help in normalising blood pressure.

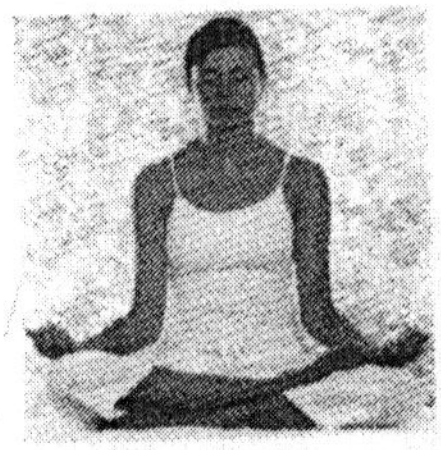

MEDITATION

The constant chanting of a silently repeated word or mantra helps to achieve relaxation by avoiding external thoughts.

REDUCTION IN BODY WEIGHT

Increased body weight can lead to hypertension, increased blood sugar & coronary blockages. Hence maintaining one's body weight is very important.

DRUGS (IF REQUIRED)

If all the above measures fail one should consult a doctor who will prescribe medicines. Medicines should never be stopped abruptly/ suddenly, as it may result in a shoot up of blood pressure which could be fatal.

General Dos and Don'ts in the treatment of High Blood pressure:

People with hypertension should avoid certain activities and situations that may raise their heart rates and blood pressure to dangerous levels. These include the following:

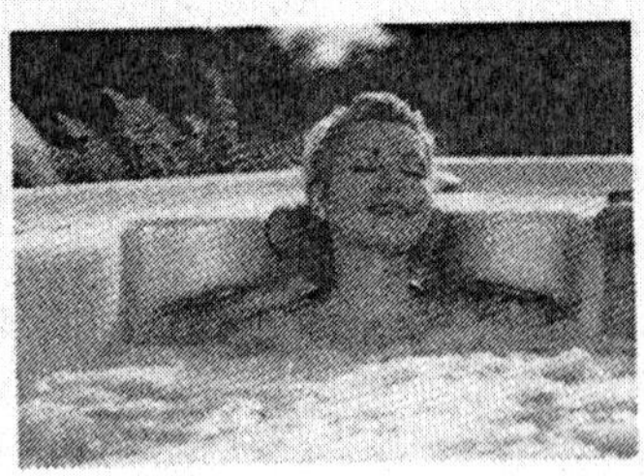

a. Saunas
b. Steam baths
c. Steam rooms
d. Heated whirlpools
e. Hot tubs
f. Very warmly heated swimming pools

If one still wants to go ahead with these activities or if you had been already doing these activities it is very important for hypertensive patients to limit the amount of time spent in these activities to less than 10 minutes, after which they should sit down out of the heat for a few minutes before standing to minimize the risk of dizziness or passing out (syncope).

Hypertensives should also be careful about using certain over-the-counter (OTC) medications that contain vasoconstrictors, which can elevate blood pressure. Such medications include:

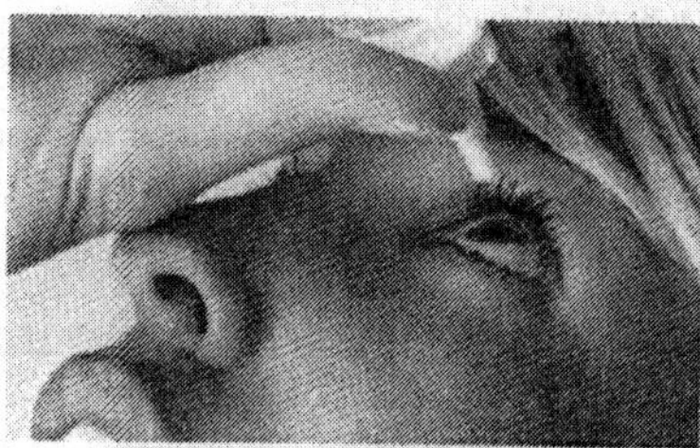

a. Eye drops
b. Cold, flu, sinus and cough medications (especially those containing decongestants)
c. Antihistamines

Hypertensives are also encouraged to follow all of their physician's orders regarding treatment, in order to prevent serious health consequences. However, patients are encouraged to discuss with their physicians any side effects or other concerns that they may have about their treatment.

❑

Chapter-4

Diet for Treatment of High Blood Pressure

1. Salt restriction & sensitivity
2. Dash Diet
3. Diet low in Fat & Cholesterol
4. Diet for weight reduction
5. High fiber
6. High anti-oxidants

There are five major aspects of diet that need to be taken care for patients with high BP and these are Salt restriction, Calorie reduction for those who are overweight, cutting down of Fat intake, high intake of Fruits and Vegetables and increased intake of Anti-oxidants. Let us consider each of them one by one.

HIGH SALT INTAKE AND HYPERTENSION

One of the major causes of high pressure is high salt or sodium intake. Salt affects blood pressure because it causes the body to retain more water. Normally, the kidneys flush the excess salt and water from the body. However, kidneys that are malfunctioning, are unable to expel them properly, which leads to fluid retention. Because the function of the kidneys is so closely tied with the body's circulatory system, changes in blood pressure will prompt the kidneys to make adjustments. If the kidneys malfunction and there is excess fluid in the system, hypertension will result.

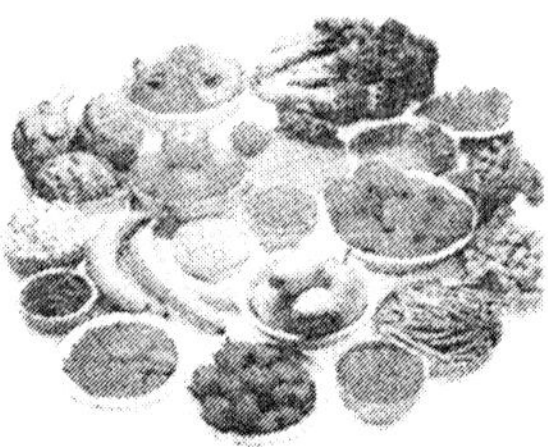

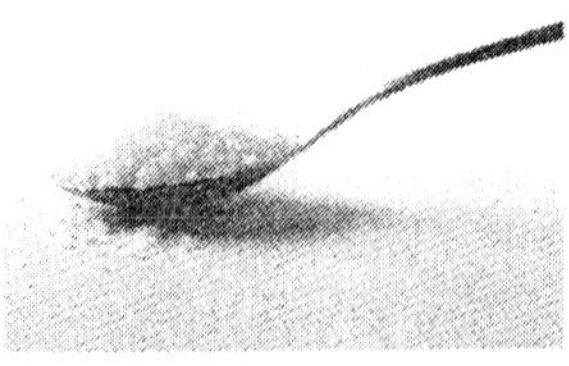

Conversely, if hypertension exists, the kidneys will slow down and excess salt and fluid will be collected in the body, adding further to the problem of hypertension .

SALT SENSITIVITY

Salt restriction may not be able to help all the patients of high blood pressure – as some people may be salt insensitive. Those who are salt sensitive usually respond to salt restriction almost immediately. The blood pressure drops down immediately. About 50% of high BP patients are salt insensitive.

To know if you are salt sensitive or not, you can do an experiment which will last for twelve days. Measure your blood pressure on all the 12 days at the same time. First 4 days take normal amount of salt, for the next 4 days cut down the salt drastically and for the last four days take extra amount of salt. If the BP goes down and up with restriction and excess intake of salt – you are salt sensitive. If the blood pressure is same all the time you are salt insensitive.

The intake of salt for a normal person is about 20-25 grams. For salt restriction we should at least look for 25% intake and cut down 75% in the diet. If the blood pressure is very high and the patients are having heart failure we can restrict the salt intake to 1 to 2 grams per day. In fact our need of sodiun in the food is just half a gram of sodium. Nowadays many low sodium salts are available in the market. LoNa salt, suffola salt belong to this category and are widely available.

Remember most of the preservatives, processed foods have excess amount of sodium. Baking soda and baking powder also have lots of sodium.

However for all the high BP patients –irrespective of their salt sensitivity salt should be restricted.

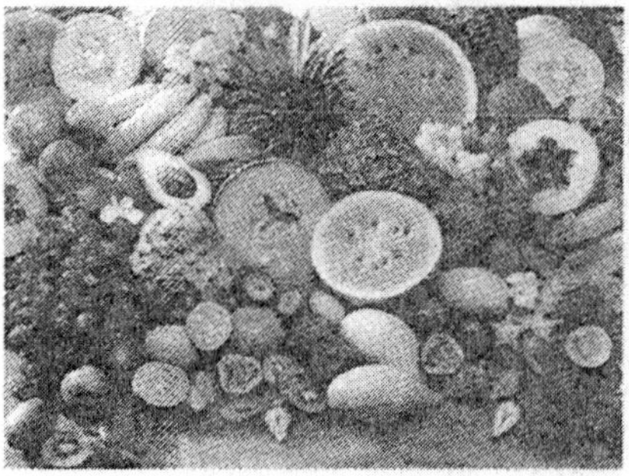

DASH DIET:

In 1997 a research study called DASH (Dietary Approaches to Stop Hypertension) was carried out in USA. About 500 patients of high BP were divided into three groups – one group took low fruits, low vegetables, excess fats and milk / milk products (Grossly unhealthy diet and an average American takes). The second group took lots of fruits and vegetables but also took excess amount of fats and milk/milk products (less healthy diet). The third group took extra fruits, extra vegetables, extra cereals and cut down intake of fats, milk/milk products (most healthy diet).

The result of the study showed that the blood pressure came down in the second group and the third group showed maximum reduction. The Dash diet analysed and showed that increased intake of Potassium, Calcium and Magnesium reduced the blood pressure in high Blood pressure patients.

All the three are present in excess in fruits, vegetables, whole grains, legumes. Green leafy vegetables and legumes contain very good amount of calcium and Magnesium.

If you want to follow DASH diet in India you should do the following:

- Have a glass of fruit juice or vegetable juice in the breakfast.
- Take some cereal (corn, wheat, whole rice) and add extra berries and slices of banana in it.
- Eat salad compulsorily in your lunch and dinner.
- Add tomato, sprouts and greens in your Sandwich or roti or rice.
- Take baked potato; vegetables made from Broccoli, cauliflower and carrots. Vegetables must be taken in plenty.
- Avoid meat, cheese and fried food.
- Have plenty of green vegetables as salads.
- Take low fat milk or curd.

DIET LOW IN CHOLESTEROL AND FATS(TRIGLYCERIDES)

Underlying heart damage or dysfunction, including atherosclerosis, or a build-up of plaque within the artery walls, may add to the increased blood force against the artery walls. The pressure of the blood through these restricted passage ways rises to account for a lack of space. Higher blood pressure can also result if there is more blood relative to the size of the blood vessel.

High BP and coronary heart disease go hand in hand. Excess amount of fats will increase chances of heart attack, increase obesity, make you prone to diabetes and will help to increase the BP indirectly.

Saaol Hypertension Control Program integrates these approaches with total restriction of any food with fat content altogether with strict vegetarian diet. Our zero oil foods are always good for high BP. We have created more than 1000 "zero oil recipes" which use no oil at all. We would recommend all those who are above the age of 18 years to stick to zero oil cooking and it will prevent development of high BP in future. All oils are triglycerides – whether they are saturated, monounsaturated or polyunsaturated. All are to be avoided.

Cholesterol is present in all animal foods, poultry and dairy products. They should be also restricted for control of high BP and atherosclerosis.

DIET FOR REDUCTION OF WEIGHT

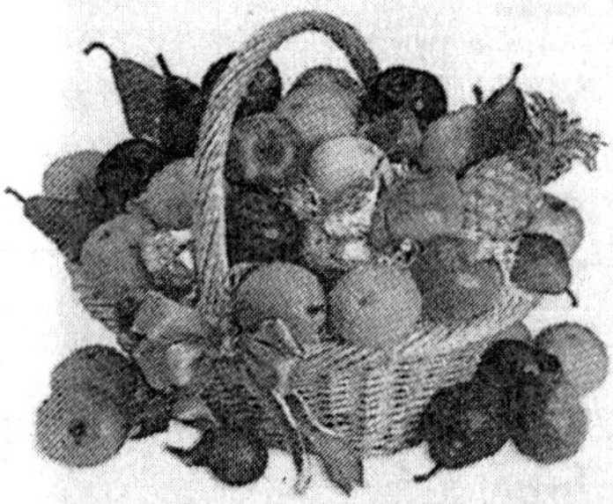

Excess body weight especially central obesity is a well known cause of high BP. The Trial of hypertension prevention (TOHP), The Trial of Non pharmacological interventions in the Elderly (TONE) and other studies have shown that 4-5 kilos of weight reduction leads to reduction of 3-4 mmHg of blood pressure. Weight reduction also increases the effects of BP lowering medicines.

One should try to reach the ideal weight if he or she wants to control high BP with least or no medications. The body weight is nowadays expressed in terms of Body Mass Index.(BMI) and ideal BMI for high BP patients is 24. The following chart gives you BMI and you should find your ideal weight for your height (your weight in KG at 24 BMI). Make your target and try to reduce 2-3 kg per month till you reach BMI 24 .

How to reduce weight?

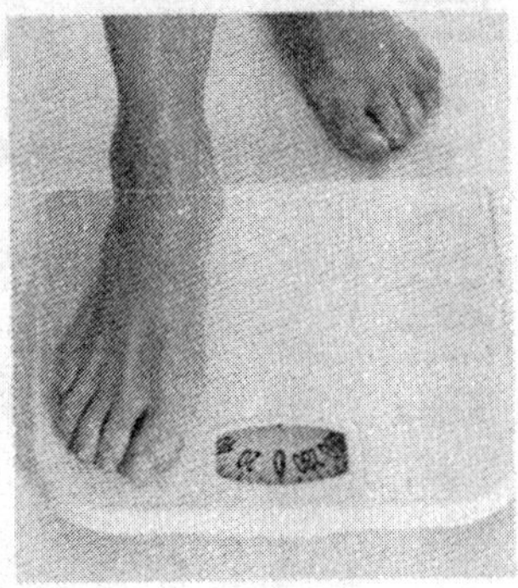

Our body needs calories (output or expenditure of calories) and we eat food which gives calories(input of calories) that run the body. Body weight will increase if the input is more than output. On the other hand, the body weight will reduce if the output is more than input. So the aim of the diet will be to modify the diet in such a way that the input of calories is reduced below the level of output. But the food should be tasty, healthy and sustainable.

FIND OUT YOUR BODY MASS INDEX

Height (Feet) ↓	Height (M) ↓	Body Weight (Kg) ↓																
4'.10'	1.47	41	44	45	48	50	52	54	56	58	61	63	65	67	69	72	74	76
4'.11"	1.50	43	45	47	49	52	54	56	58	60	63	65	67	69	72	74	76	78
5'.0"	1.52	44	46	49	51	54	56	58	60	63	65	67	69	72	74	76	79	81
5'.1"	1.55	45	48	50	53	55	58	60	62	65	67	69	72	74	77	79	82	84
5'.2"	1.57	47	49	52	54	57	59	62	64	67	69	72	74	77	79	82	84	87
5'.3"	1.60	49	51	54	56	59	61	64	66	69	72	74	77	79	82	84	87	89
5'.4"	1.62	50	53	55	58	61	64	66	68	71	74	77	79	82	84	87	89	93
5'.5"	1.65	52	54	57	60	63	65	68	71	74	76	79	82	84	87	90	93	95
5'.6"	1.68	54	56	59	62	64	67	70	73	76	78	81	84	87	90	93	95	98
5'.7"	1.70	55	58	61	64	66	69	72	75	78	81	84	87	90	93	96	99	101
5'.8"	1.72	57	59	63	65	68	72	74	78	80	84	86	89	92	95	98	101	104
5'.9"	1.75	58	61	64	68	70	74	77	80	83	86	89	92	95	98	101	104	107
5'.10"	1.78	60	63	66	69	73	76	79	82	85	88	92	95	98	101	104	107	110
5'.11	1.80	62	65	68	71	75	78	81	84	88	91	94	98	101	104	107	110	114
6'.0"	1.83	64	67	70	74	77	80	84	87	90	94	97	100	104	107	110	114	117
6'.1"	1.85	65	68	72	75	79	83	86	89	93	96	99	103	107	110	114	117	120
6'.2"	1.88	67	70	74	78	81	84	88	92	95	99	102	106	109	113	116	120	123
6'.3"	1.90	69	73	76	80	84	87	91	94	98	102	105	109	113	116	120	123	127
6'.4"	1.93	71	74	78	82	86	89	93	97	100	104	108	112	115	119	123	127	130
BMI →		19	20	21	22	23	24	25	26	27	28	29	30	31	32	33	34	35
		← Under Weight →			← Normal →				← Over Weight →				← Obesity →					

Nutrients which provide input

Man needs a wide range of nutrients to perform various functions in the body and to lead a healthy life. The nutrients include carbohydrates, proteins, fats, vitamins, minerals, water and fiber. Each of the calorie giving foods give us calories and they are as follows:

Carbohydrates	:	4 calories per gram.
Proteins	:	4 calories per gram.
Fats	:	9 calories per gram.

Vitamins and minerals do not yield energy, but they play a very important role in regulating the metabolic activities of the body. Since a man derives all the nutrients he needs through the diet he eats, his diet must be well balanced to provide all the nutrients in proper proportions. Fiber and water also do not give any calories – but play an important role in the maintenance of health.

So, our body's need for calories come from Carbohydrates (cereals, sugar, fruits and Vegetables), proteins (legumes and pulses, milk and animal foods) and fats (all oils, butter, cream, cheese etc).

Body's expenditure or Output of Calories

For every activity that we do the body needs calories. The following chart shows how many calories do we require per minute. A sedentary man – who does very little physical exertion- needs about 1600 calories in total in a day. These calories will come from the calorie foods namely – the Carbohydrates , proteins and fats.

ACTIVITY	ENERGY EXP.
Sleeping	0.5 c/minute
Reading	1.4 c/minute
Eating	1.8 c/minute
Conversing	1.8 c/minute
Sitting / Writing	2.0 c/minute
Driving a car	2.1 c/minute
Standing	2.2 c/minute
Casual walking	4-5 c/minute
Brisk walking	6-8 c/minute
Jogging	7-9 c/minute
Playing football	7-10 c/minute
Running	10-12 c/minute

Usual diet of a well to do Indian

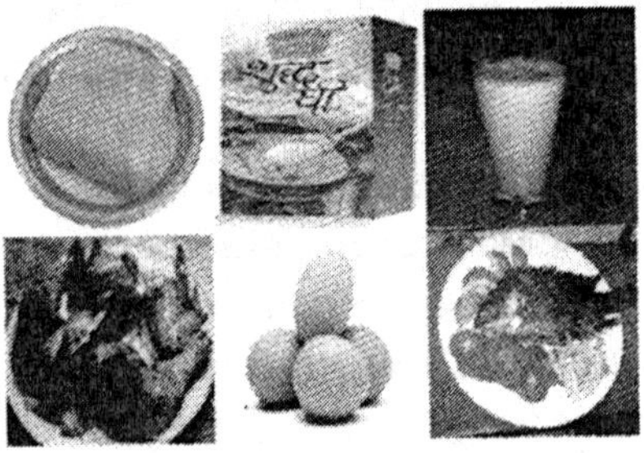

An ideal Indian from upper or upper middle socio-economic class usually consumes lots of fats and high calorie carbohydrates. About 40-50% calories come from Fats and 40-50% come from carbohydrates. About 10-20% calories are contributed by the proteins. The total input usually exceeds the output.

Food for reducing weight

To reduce calories in the diet the first and the foremost thing to do is cut down the fats in the food. For this we advice cutting down all the fatty foods like fried food, dry foods, cheese, butter, chocolates and ice creams. For cooking, the food we advice **" Zero oil Cooking"**. Remember that one gram of fat has 9 calories and it is the fats which lead to obesity.

In the carbohydrates also we want them to eat more salads, vegetables and fruits to provide more filling fibers along with the carbohydrates. They should take sugar and cereals in moderation or in low quantity till they want to lose weight.

Food items that are to be taken and avoided for reduction of weight

Foods to be avoided

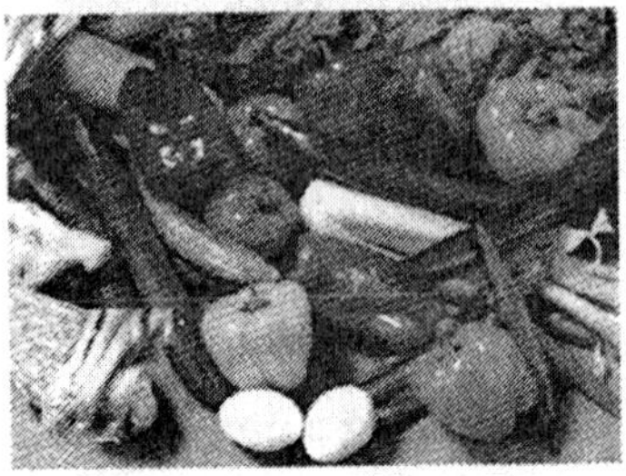

1. Milk (full cream) and its Products
2. Cheese and butter
3. All fried foods and farsans
4. All kinds of high fat Non-vegetarian items
5. Chocolates and Ice creams
6. Nuts and Dry fruits
7. Sweets (Mithai)
8. Oil (All types of oils)
9. Cold Drinks (Sheetal Pay).

Foods that are Moderately Restricted

1. Brown Bread & White Bread (Double Roti)
2. Chapati, Roti (Wheat)

3. Rice (Chawal)
4. Vermicelli (Sewai)
5. Bajra (Bajra)
6. Jowar
7. Maize (Makka)
8. Peas (Dry) (Matar Sukha)
9. Potato, Sweet Potato (Shakarkandi), Arvi
10. Jaggery (Gur)
11. Cane Sugar (Chini)
12. Banana (Ripe) (Kela)
13. Mango.
14. Thick Dal

Foods that can be Consumed Freely

1. Bathua Leaves (Bathua Sag)
2. Spinach (Palak)
3. Radish Leaves (Mooli ka Saag)
4. Cabbage (Patta Gobhi)
5. Amaranth (Cholai Saag)
6. Carrot Leaves (Gajar Saag)
7. Radish Leaves (Muli ka Saag)
8. Calocasia Leaves (Arvi ka Saag)
9. Drumstick (Saijan)
10. Fenugreek (Methi Saag)
11. Lettuce (Salad leaves)
12. Mint (Pudina)
13. Mustard Leaves (Sarson Saag)
14. Yam, ordinary (Jimikand)
15. Carrot (Gajar)
16. Onion (Pyaj)
17. White Radish (Safed Mooli)
18. Garlic
19. Ginger
20. Beans (Sem)
21. Brinjal (Baigan)
22. Cucumber (Kheera)
23. French Beans (Bakla)
24. Lotus stem (Dry) (Kamal Gatta)
25. Parwar (Parwal)

26. Pumpkin (Kaddu)
27. Lady-finger (Bhindi)
28. Tinda (Tinda)
29. Tomato (Tamatar)
30. Bottle Guord (Ghia)
31. Turai
32. Capsicum (Shimla Mirch)
33. Kakri
34. Mushrooms
35. Apple (Seb)
36. Guava (Amrood)
37. Lemon (Nimbu)
38. Mousami
39. Orange (Santara)
40. Melon water (Tarbooj)
41. Papaya (Ripe Papita)
42. Pina Apple (Ananas)
43. Tomato Ripe
44. Musk Melon (Kharbooza)

DIET FOR HIGH FIBER AND ANTI OXIDANTS

(Eat plenty of fruits, vegetables and cereals)

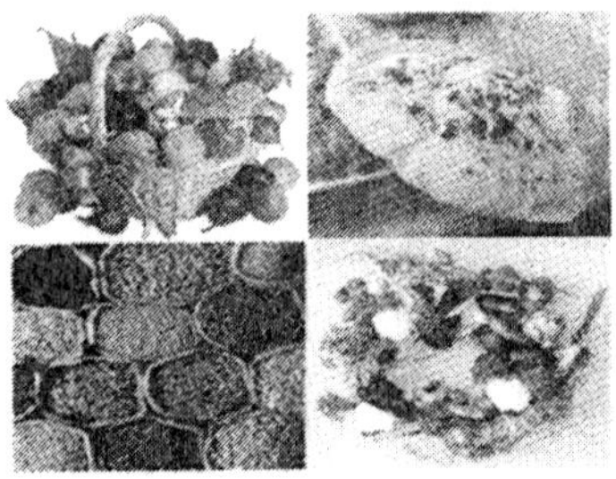

Foods that have high content of fiber has been shown to reduce the blood pressure. Fibers are also called roughage and are never absorbed from the intestine. High fiber foods are also low in calories and suit obese high BP patients.

Anti oxidants are vitamins and micro nutrients - which also help to prevent atherosclerosis and thus indirectly help to reduce high Blood pressure. These vitamins called Vitamin A, Vitamin C and Vitamin E and chemicals called cromium, zinc , copper, manganese, molybdenum are supposed to prevent hardening of the arteries and retard ageing as well.

High BP patients must increase the intake of foods which have fibers and antioxidants.

❑

Chapter-5

Stress Management to control High Blood Pressure

As has been already discussed stress management is the major factor that can help reduction of High Blood pressure. All of us know that our blood pressure rises immediately as soon as we increase our stress or become angry. Whenever we are under pressure from anywhere the blood pressure shoots up. The opposite also hold good. When you relax the blood pressure goes down. People are so aware of these facts that whenever I measure the pressure of someone and find it more – immediately the patient would reply –"Sir, I have just come after 1 hour of driving. This stress has increased the BP today. At home my BP just remains normal."

If you see the literal meaning of Hypertension – it means "excess stress".

a. Training of the Rational Brain and Taming our Emotional mind.
b. Understanding stress and its effects on our life.
c. Identifying the role of our surroundings in production of stress and how to handle these external factors.
d. Understanding our attitude, desires, reactions, wants and the mindset. Modification of our mindset.
e. Avoiding the overloads of life.
f. Balancing the sectors of our life.
g. Release and management of stress.
h. Improving the way we speak.

Whenever stress is produced a chemical called adrenaline is released into our blood along with a chemical called Cortisol. These two are responsible for Stress Reaction – the response of the body to stressful inputs.

1. RATIONAL AND EMOTIONAL BRAIN

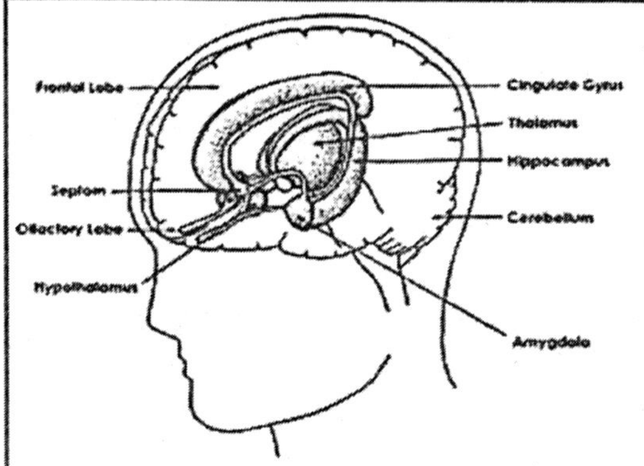

The limbic system, or animal brain

Stress is a phenomenon produced in the brain and thus we should discuss the structure of the brain before going further on management of stress. From functional point of view ,our brain has two components – one the **Rational Brain** and the second – **the Emotional Brain.** The rational brain is called the Cerebral cortex and is responsible for all our day- to-day actions, thinking, learning, speech, memory, understanding of the surroundings. The emotional brain is called the Limbic Cortex and is responsible for all out emotional unsteadiness. Emotional brain contributes largely to our anger, irritations, greed, jealousy and so on.

The technique of stress management that I would describe will involve **"training of the Rational Brain and taming of the Emotional Brain"**. The beauty is that the rational brain would understand all the logic, would analyse the cause and effects of stress in our life. But the emotional brain does not understand logic – it needs to be tamed by yoga and meditation.

Lets feed the Rational mind with more information on stress and its management.

2. UNDERSTANDING STRESS AND ITS EFFECTS ON OUR LIFE

Definition of Stress

Stress is a universal word which is being used by just about anyone, everywhere you go. A clear cut definition has not been evolved yet. Try defining it yourself and see the kind of difficulties you face!

The medical science describes stress as a specific response of the body to all nonspecific demands be it physical or psychological, be it threatened or actual — the response being the secretion of ACTH and cortisol (these are two stress induced hormones). Secretion of two other hormones stimulated by stress are Adrenaline and Non Adrenaline.

A more practical definition of stress may be put as "When the problem presented by every day life exceeds your resources for coping with them you feel stressed." But we must remember that stress cannot be imposed solely by external demands or problems but can also be generated from within, that is internally by our hopes, fears, expectations and beliefs.

How to identify a stressed person?

A good number of individuals I have met over the years do not agree that they are stressed. They simply cannot accept the fact that they have problems because they have not been observant or have not tried to understand their responsibilities in different aspects of their lives. The success with money and a short lasting increased ego sometimes does not allow them to concede.

The following are some distinguishing features of excessive stress:

Physical symptoms:

1. Tensed muscles (shoulder ache, back ache)
2. Irregular breathing
3. Dry mouth
4. Sweaty palms
5. Cold fingers
6. Knots in the stomach
7. Shaky hands
8. Frequency of urination

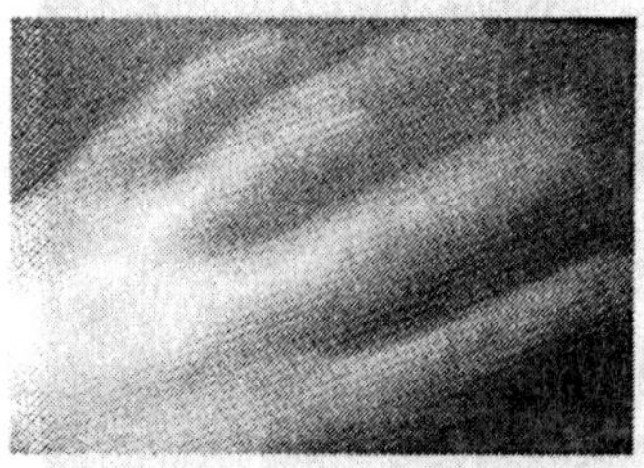

Behavioral symptoms:

1. Smoking
2. Tobacco consumption (e.g. Gutka)
3. Repeated stimulant intake (e.g. tea,coffee)
4. Increased alcohol consumption
5. Nail biting, knee jingling, hair pulling
6. Reckless driving
7. Social withdrawal
8. Disinterested look.

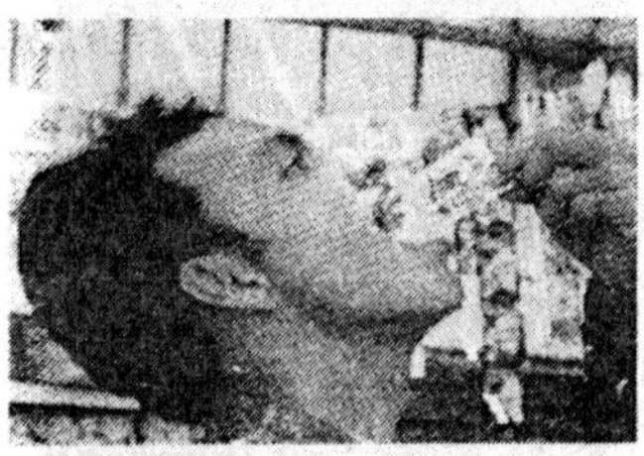

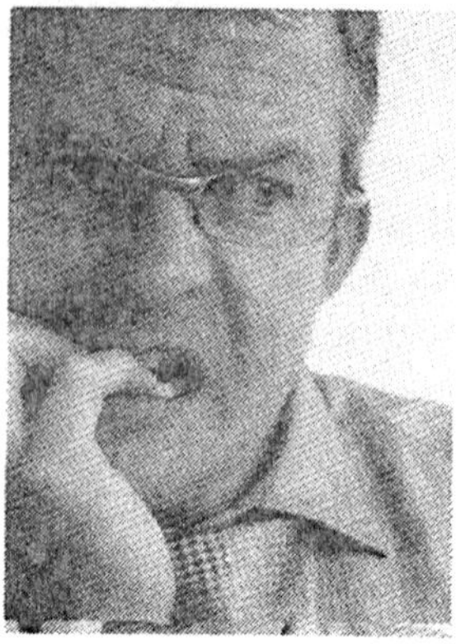

Emotional Symptoms:

1. Irritability
2. Short temper
3. Undue haste
4. State of anxiety
5. Feeling of depression
6. Irrational fear
7. Feeling of insecurity
8. Undue aggression
9. Sleeplessness
10. Bad dreams.

Cognitive symptoms:

1. Loss of sense of humor
2. Loss of memory
3. Forgetfulness
4. Loss of common sense
5. Loss of clarity of thinking
6. Indecisiveness
7. Undue fear
8. Black and white thoughts.

Well, one or more of the above may be your problem or problems of people you associate with. Beware, they tend to bother you more on the days you are most stressed and disappear on days when you are relaxed and not stressed.

Mentioned below are some of the changes produced by the human body in response to stress. You will shortly observe that most of these responses of the human body to stress's are harmful to the individual, his personal, social and professional life.

Effects of stress on our body:

1. Heart rate increases
2. Blood pressure increases
3. Muscle tension increases
4. G.S.R. decreases
5. Respiratory rate increases
6. Oxygen consumption increases
7. Spasm of arteries
8. S. Cortisol increases

9. S. Catecholamines/adrenalin increases
10. Blood sugar increases
11. Serum cholesterol increases
12. Acid in stomach increases
13. Blood clotting increases
14. Drying of saliva
15. Bowel and bladder tone decreases

3. STRESS AND DISEASES

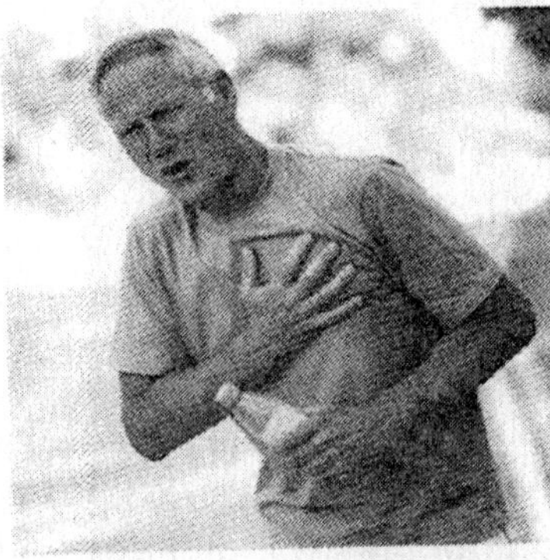

Modern science till some years ago, did not attribute stress to the creation of diseases. High blood pressure, heart disease, peptic ulcer are very common in highly placed executives and not so in a moderately satisfied earning individual or native villager. This interesting finding can only be explained on the basis of severe stress that the former experiences.

In the last few decades a series of epidemiological studies and observations have proved that some very common diseases are a direct result of excessive stress. They are now grouped as psychosomatic diseases.

A list of these common diseases follows:

1. High blood pressure
2. Angina or chest pain
3. Heart attacks (Myocardial infarction or MI)
4. Tension headache's
5. Migraine
6. Backache
7. Shoulder ache
8. Spondylosis
9. Palpitation
10. Allergies
11. Asthma
12. Chronic fatigue and lethargy
13. Anxiety state
14. Phobias

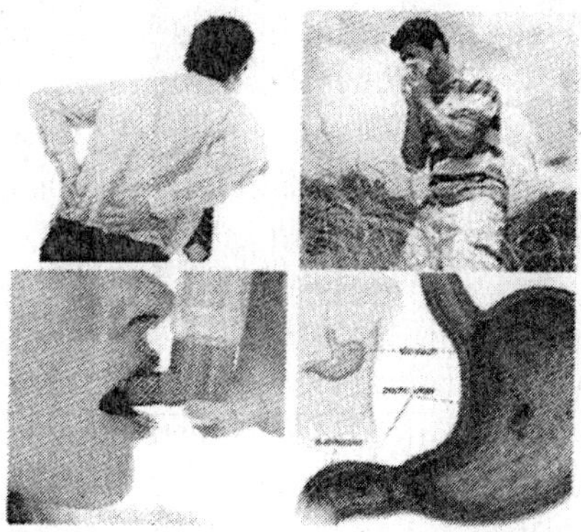

15. Insomnia
16. Depression
17. Irritable bowel syndrome (IBS)
18. Peptic ulcer
19. Pre-menstrual syndrome in females.

Do you suffer from any of them? Be honest with yourself and try to identify and understand your problems and their proportions, this will help you to clearly define a solution for them.

4. THE PRODUCTION OF STRESS

"Stress is produced when things do not happen the way we want". Please read this sentence few times and try to understand the meaning. In stress production two factors work – one is what is happening and the second is what we want. If we can match both of them – stress will not be produced and happiness will result.

What is happening is present in our surrounding and are called External Stressors. What I want is inside the brain. This can be called internal factor or Mindset. Let us understand both.

1. External factors: I would like to call it the stressor. I shall give a list of examples of possible stresses. Please identify them. An external stressor has almost equal contribution to stress. Even recognition of these is of great help in the management of stress.

2. Internal factors: This is the result of our previous experiences, training, values and expectations. Our beliefs, hopes, attitude, aspirations influence the internal factor. This can also be called "MINDSET" . These values keep on changing slowly over the years in order to adjust to our changing surroundings. Any stagnation or fast change in the internal factors make a person more susceptible to stress.

Copying with Stress Production

Development of Coping Ability

Coping with stress is an innate ability of our body and mind in combination. We need to perceive the stress - handle the external and internal factors in proper way.

The ability of the person in this regard remains dormant or un-utilized most often. Many people have a misdirected ability. This is where training counts. If the coping ability is good, the perceived stress can be minimized or eliminated. On the other hand, a bad coping ability can worsen the stress experienced. To reduce stress production we have to match both the external as well as internal factors (mind set).

5. HANDLING OF YOUR EXTERNAL FACTORS

Examples of the External Stressors

Social & Family

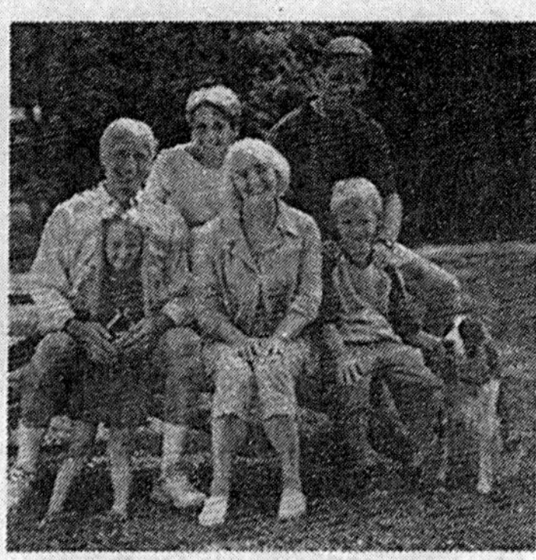

1. High unrealistic expectations.
2. Indifferent to spouse.
3. Lack of communication with family members.
4. Recurrent financial problems.
5. Different values and priorities.
6. Different sleeping patterns.
7. Ugly or very beautiful wife/ husband.
8. Differences about work sharing.
9. Spouse who talks too much.
10. Spouse/member who is unnecessarily rude.
11. Death/Illness of a family member.
12. Frequent guests.
13. Unfaithfulness.
14. Relatives with unreasonable expectations.
15. Difficult neighbours.

Occupation

1. Change-requiring new skills.
2. Boss with abusive communication style.
3. Subordinates who are incompetent.
4. Colleagues who do not co-operate.
5. Poor administration.
6. Bureaucracy.
7. Numerous deadlines.
8. Socialization during work
9. Lack of control over work environment
10. Lack of feedback from the top or bottom
11. Inadequate rewards
12. Time and work overload
13. Unclear authority
14. Long working hours
15. No holidays.

Political

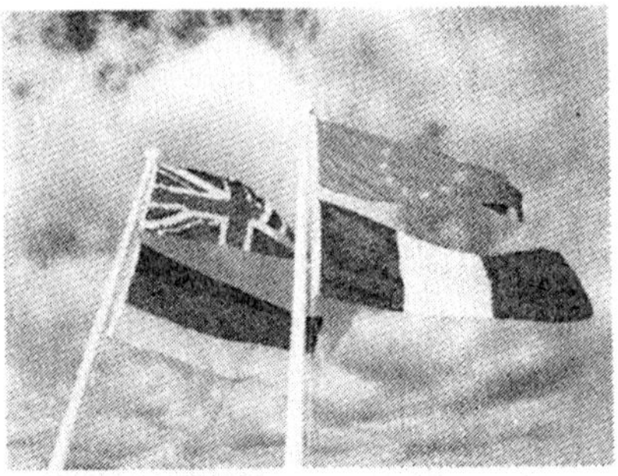

1. Unsteady political scenario
2. Corrupt ministers of parliament
3. Corrupt or un co-operative bureaucrats
4. Lack of leadership
5. Dictatorship
6. Strikes
7. International tension
8. Unfulfilled promises
9. Wrong media coverage
10. Industrial policy
11. Politicizing of religion
12. Repeated demonstrations of violence
13. Incompetent ministers
14. Criminals in Politics
15. Unfair elections.

Ecology

1. Increasing pollution
2. Deforestation
3. Urban crowding
4. Unplanned cities and towns
5. Adulteration of food
6. Loss of natural resources
7. Water pollution
8. Over industrialization
9. Radiation hazard
10. Noise pollution
11. Industrial accidents
12. Nuclear arms race
13. Ozone layer depletion
14. Extinction of rare animals
15. Green house effects.

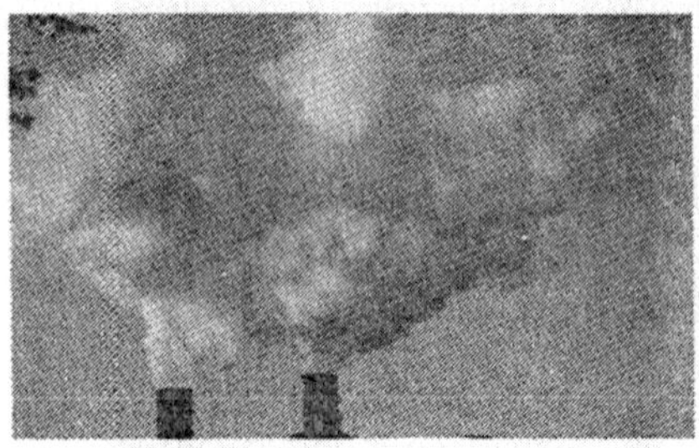

Physical & Psychological

1. Extreme hot or cold atmosphere
2. Dress - too tight or loose

3. Noisy surroundings at work/home
4. Uncomfortable chairs
5. Poor lighting and ventilation
6. Continuous bending, standing
7. Excessive eye strain
8. Lack of cleanliness
9. Lack of regards for safety regulations
10. Sarcastic remarks
11. Politics in office
12. Hostile atmosphere
13. Isolated atmosphere
14. Over crowded environment
15. People who create problems

Moral Values / Social change

1. Generation gap
2. Lack of morality
3. Class discrimination
4. Permissiveness/openness
5. Human rights violation
6. Violence
7. Movies, TV, books giving wrong messages
8. Social isolation
9. Housing shortage
10. Disharmony with the neighbours
11. Changed feelings about parents and teachers
12. Unfair trade or practice
13. Undependable friends and relatives
14. Social outcasts
15. Plight of sick, poor or old.

Economic

1. Inflation
2. Slow economic growth
3. Water crisis
4. Power shortage
5. Union power
6. Reduced productivity
7. Export - import gap

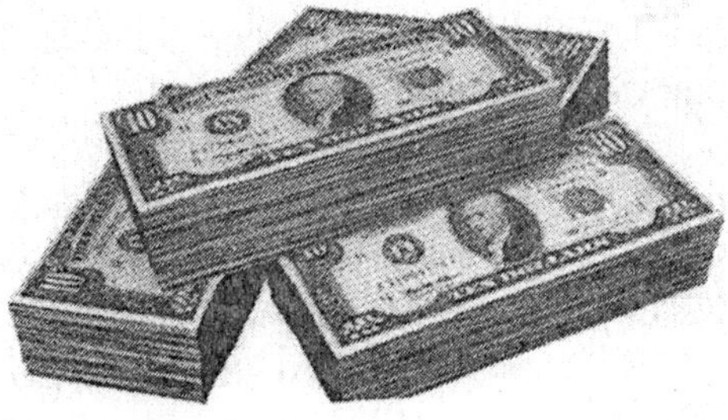

8. Rich - poor gap
9. Excessive price of land and houses
10. Rising interest rates
11. Lack of cash flow
12. Bureaucracy in financial institutions
13. Cut in public expenditure
14. Over population and competitions for jobs
15. Fast changing technology.

What to do about External factors:

We are always surrounded by these external factors and throughout the day we need to interact with them. We need to know how to handle them. Not all of them will be handled similarly. It is similar to a cricket match. You are a batsman and are getting different kinds of balls. For each of them you need to have different shots. Let us see what are the possibilities.

1.Identify : There are so many external stressors we just need to identify and the stress production will go down. It may be that you stay in Delhi and there is excess traffic. You identify that it is a important city and more people stay here and they have so many cars. So, the traffic will be excess. Your rational brain will immediately understand and stress production will become less. There are so many factors in our surrounding which only needs identification and stress from that will go away.

2. Modify: Some of the external stressors can be modified. You are late for your work every day. You could identify that there is so much of work to be done in the morning and you would be running short of time. Modify your time of getting up. Stop reading newspaper in the morning. Now your problem is solved.

3. Avoid: Many external stressors can be avoided. The day you drink alcohol there is a fight with your wife. So, avoid alcohol. There is a neighbour who is very difficult – you start avoiding him. Your stress is now not produced.

4. Accept: Some of the external factors cannot be avoided or modified. They have to be accepted. It may be your spouse's behavior, your aging, your prime minister, your city, rainy season. Just try to make a list of such things where you should not react but only accept.

5. Do not get involved: There are many things which really do not affect you and still you get involved. Let it happen. You should not try to poke your nose into it. It may be the marriage of one of your relatives with someone you will not like. It may be the erratic actions of a politician which does not really affect you. Do not take stress. It may be the way that your neighbours dress. Just be indifferent.

6. Fight: There are situations where you may need to fight. If the stake is high you need to fight. Someone is snatching your property worth crores, you have to fight.

6. MINDSET AND ITS HANDLING:

Understanding Mindset

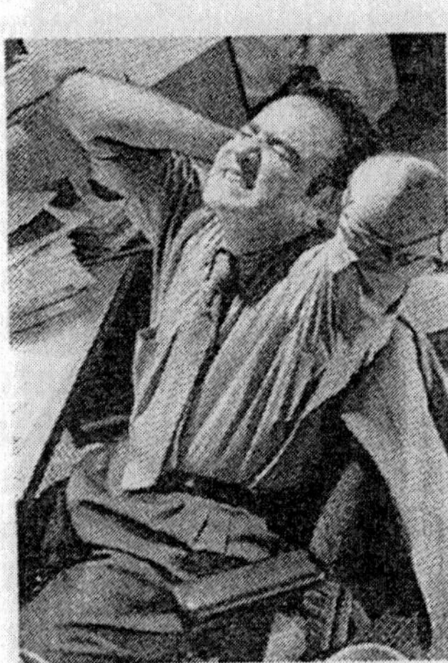

Mindset or internal factors is what you want. When we are born the brain is blank. It has no feeling of good or bad, no preferences, it has no likes and dislikes, but gradually we start feeding the mind with facts and information. Starting from the age of one or two years our mind starts learning. The cues are taken from the surroundings- from what you see, hear and feel. You start learning a particular language – you start liking that language. You learn Bengali, you like Bengali. You learn Tamil and start liking it. You like a particular food – you start loving it. If you start eating fish and love it, you will feel stressed if you do not get it. On the other hand someone who has not eaten fish – does not want to have fish. This is called Mindset. This is your internal conditioning or factor.

All of us have this mindset developed over the years. This may be the person you like or dislike, food you like or dislike. It may be anything ranging from your dress, language, subject of learning, accuracy about work, feeling about money, idea about relationship, morality. There are thousands of likes and dislikes developed in every one's mind.

Stress is produced when the external factors or happenings do not match your mindset. We have already learnt about what to do about external stressors like (identify, modify, avoid, accept, do not get involved, fight- are some of the choices). Now let us understand what can we do to modify or change our mindset. Let our rational mind - which understands logic – analyse it.

Handling of the mindset

Three major things are to be understood for modification of our mind set. These are – change with time, anekant and that society is based on give and take. Appreciating these three will make your mind malleable.

Change with time: Our mindsets have been set when we were younger – may be few years back or even few months back, but now things have changed. Fashions have changed, society has changed, your status has changed, your education level has changed, the composition of family has changed. You also need to change. You now have high blood pressure – you need to change some foods which you used to like. Someone has cheated you – you cannot now trust him. He was a friend – now you need to make some changes in your mind. Someone has died – your mind has to now start accepting that all is not the same. Reset your mind with changing time and environment. All of us make such changes. You also have to do this.

Theory of Anekant: This theory comes from the ancient scriptures of Agam written in Pali language. But its application in our present life is so logical. *"Anek"* means many. *"Anekant"* says everyone has a different mindset. About same things many different people will have different opinion. Depending on the surrounding they grow the mindsets are different. A Chinese likes Chinese language and you may like Hindi. The food choices will be different for the husband and wife. The thinking will also be different. The likes and dislikes will be different. The more you understand Anekant – the more your interpersonal relationship will change. You will be able to appreciate the behavior of your friends, relatives, employees, employers, children, spouse or even of unknown persons. Your stress production from others behavior will drastically reduce.

Society is based on Give and take: This is another theory that can change your stress production. Suppose there are two people who have two different mindsets (say liking and dislikes) and they have to live together. Now unless they adjust with each other the group will not survive. Other wise they will keep on fighting with each other. It is ideal that these adjustments must come from both the parties. Similarly in our society so many people live with each other. They will co-exist better and without a lot of stress if they appreciate and apply this theory of "Give and Take".

7. PRESSURES (OVERLOADS) OF LIFE

Stress has increased tremendously in our life in the last fifty years. With stress has increased the lifestyle related diseases including high blood pressure. The more you are stressed the more the blood pressure rises. Once I met a philosopher and enquired about the causes of these increasing stresses – he explained to me five major overloads. These overloads are Work overload, Time overload, Information overload, Requirement overload and lastly Illness overload. Let us consider them one by one.

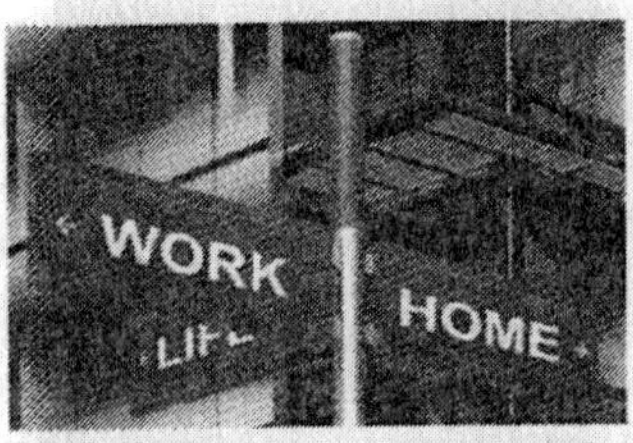

Work Pressure (Overload): In our life we now have to work much more than we previously used to do. The families have become nuclear and work share has gone up. Government and private offices are demanding more work from you. You also want to earn more, do more business – so more hours have to be spent. People are working 10-16 hours in the whole of the day. Work is on from morning 5 AM to 11PM in the night. Even sleeping time has to be reduced in many. Thus the stress is more.

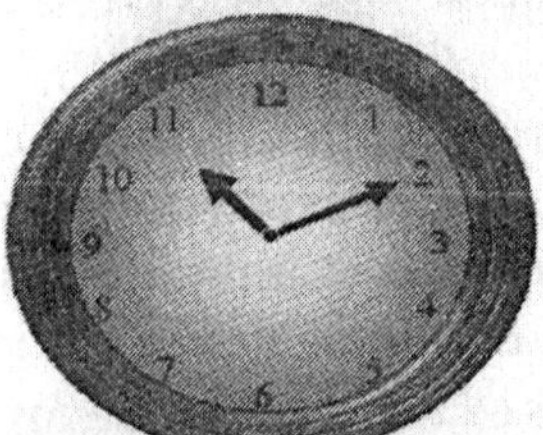

Time Pressure (Overload): Consider yourself pressed for time. You have to reach for an important meeting and you are stuck in a traffic jam. You have to catch a train or flight and you are delayed. The Blood pressure will surely go up. This is happening in lives of every busy man or woman who has to work more to survive or to excel. Work has increased but time available to everyone is same. You have to manage within that time. The travel time has gone up, you are facing traffic delays, there are so many places where you are losing time. You are part of a so called Rat race and you can't give up.

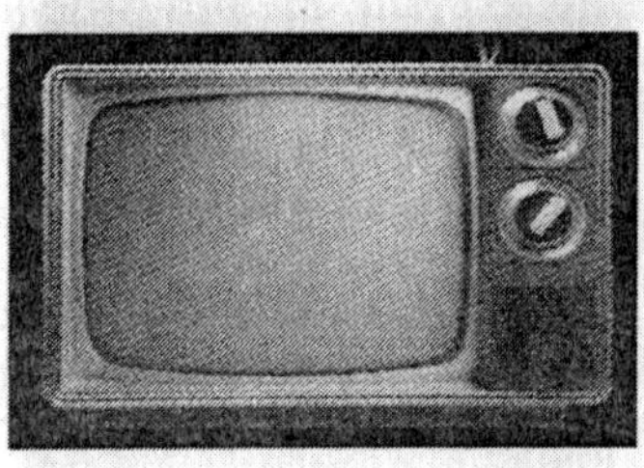

Information Pressure (Overload): Our mind is very small if you consider the amount of knowledge and information that is available. Books are full of information, TVs are full of information, newspapers and magazines are full of information, internet is full of information. Your success depends on how much information you can gather or handle. This is a modern era of information technology. Knowledge is money. There is an explosion of information. Teacher has to know more; doctors, advocates, scientists, executives, businessmen all have to know more. So, there is excessive load on the brain.

Requirement Pressure (Overload): This stems from our desire to acquire more. This may often turn up to be the most important cause of stress and in turn of High Blood Presuure. There is also a pressure from other family members to acquire more. More things are required to lead life now. The mind is seeing so many possibilities that there is a urge to buy more. The TV, the magazines, the newspapers are full of advertisements of things which can be bought. This is more so with the younger generation but modern adults are now also in the same boat. We need more clothes, more shoes, more watches, more gadgets, more TVs, more ornaments, more facilities. Inability to get them increases our stress. To fulfill these requirements we need to work more and also suffer from time overload. Many of us resort to unfair means to earn money. All these lead to excess stress. To reduce this requirement overload we should learn to make life simple, our desires have to be reined. We must learn to distinguish between "Need to have and Nice to have". We should try to get the needs and cut down the things from the list of "Nice to have". This is why many people with little money are happier than many with lot of money.

Illness Pressure (Overload): Our body has been built in such a way that it can last for 100 years without illness. But if we do not give it ideal food, ideal environment, good maintenance, optimum physical exercise – it starts getting diseased. Some diseases are acquired from the environment but most of the common diseases of the mankind today are lifestyle related. Our health is in real sense our wealth. If health is lost – all the overloads will be created. You stop enjoying life. This is when prevention is required. For this you need to spend some time, acquire some health related education and undergo certain tests from time to time. Health problems really shoot up our stresses.

8. BALANCING THE STRESS SECTORS OF LIFE:

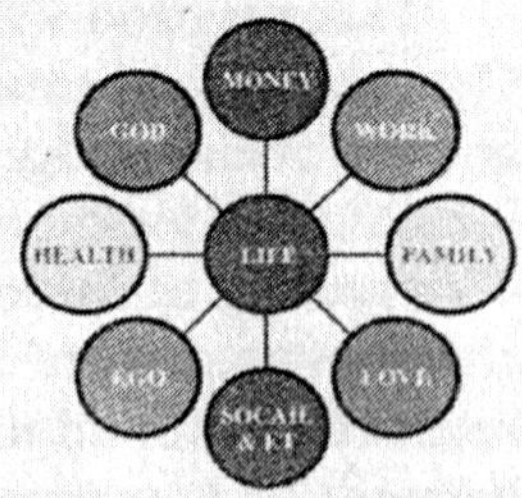

Our life is multi dimensional. Some major sectors govern our stresses from many angles. These are called Sectors of life. Any difficulties in any of the sectors can lead to excessive stress in our life. It affects the brain and thus leads to secretion of adrenaline. Let us consider each of these sectors.

Money sector: If you talk of practicality of life – money has evolved as the most important stress buster and creator also. Money is required for every activity in life. You get up from the bed in the morning and switch on the light – you need to pay for it. You want to brush your teeth – you need money to buy tooth brush and tooth paste. You want to take a bath – you need water, soap, shampoo, you need money to buy them. You want to have breakfast, wear clothes, travel to your work – for everything you need to pay money. So if money is in short supply your stress is going to be very high. So you need to earn and have money to keep you stress free throughout the day. But everyone earns money or have a source of money – why should they have stress from money? The answer is shortage of money. If the expenditure is more than income that money really bites. To keep the money sector happy you must either cut down the expenditure or increase the income. If the income is fixed - cut down your needs and urge to have more. You should also be self sufficient – not dependent on anyone for your money – your stress from money sector will go further down.

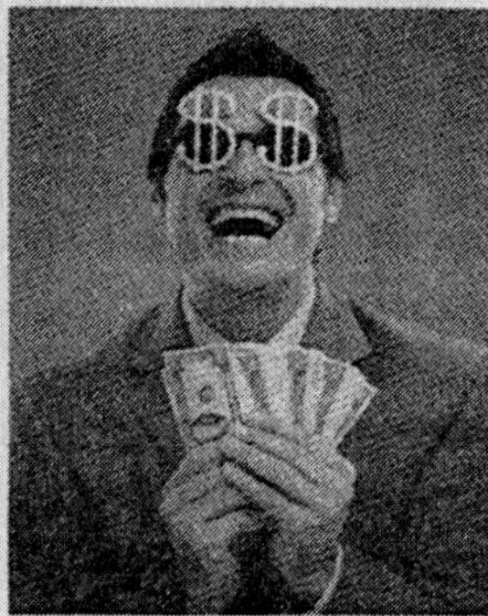

Work sector:. Besides sleeping, eating, and daily chores all of us do something by profession. Some one may be an executive, businessman, doctor, engineer, teacher or a housewife. The question is which profession is less stressful and which is highly stressful. People usually have a tendency to blame their profession for their stresses. This is not true. A profession gives stress only when you don't like it. If you love your profession, enjoy it – it gives a lot of comfort, satisfaction and happiness. So, the rule is start liking the profession that you are in. If you do not like it – change your profession to something that you love.

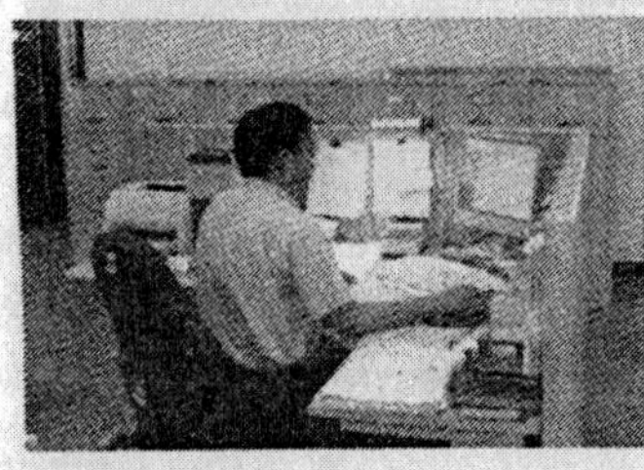

Family Sector: Many people are comfortable with their money and profession – but are stressed because of their family problems. Interpersonal relationships amongst the members of the family – if not

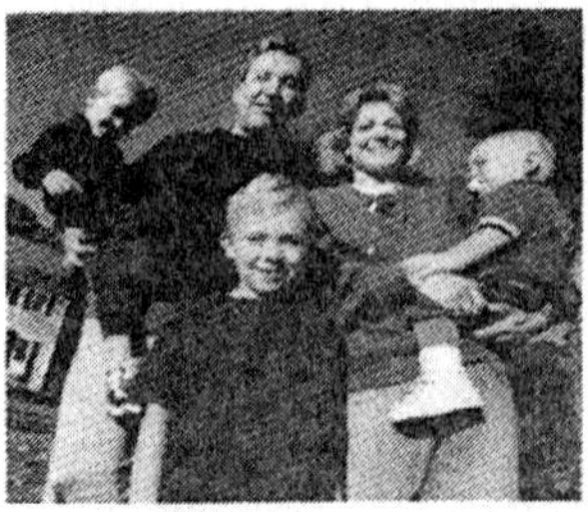

good – can be a source of continuous stress. The expectations from each other are not met. So there is tension. To improve the family tensions and stresses you should try to find out what are the interests of each of the family members and start taking efforts to encourage them in their interests. If a husband knows the likings of the wife and the wife understands what gives pleasure to the husband and both of them encourage each other in their interests – family can be a heaven. If the son and father, brother and sister, mother and son start doing the same the family will be an ideal place to enjoy. In the family remember to help each other whole heartedly, – when one is in problem, be it health or profession.

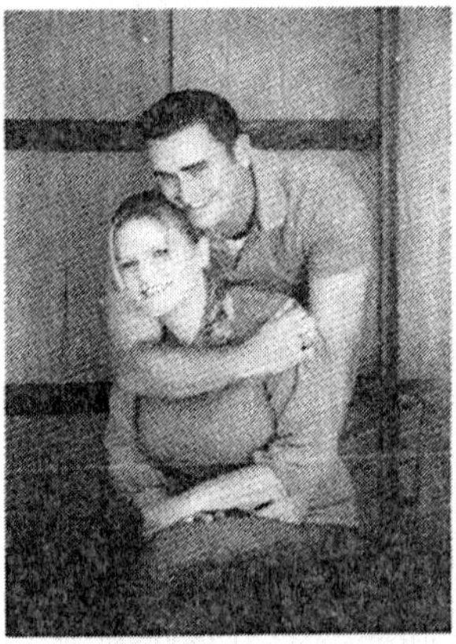

Love sector: Love or emotional support from people around us gives us a lot of happiness and removes the stresses of insecurity. In our materialistic and busy life people become more self centered and try to solve only their own problems. Other's problems do not appear so important. We have no time for others. This leads to a lot of insecurity. You remain alone and feel emotionally left out. People of the west are already feeling this lack of emotional support from their children, spouse or friends. This is also happening in India. To improve your love sector, you should try to help people without any expectations from them. The rule is to give and forget. Don't expect anything back. But if someone has helped you please always try to return their favour. Try doing this every day and you will know that lot of people feel for you, love you, try to give you back some of the love you gave them.

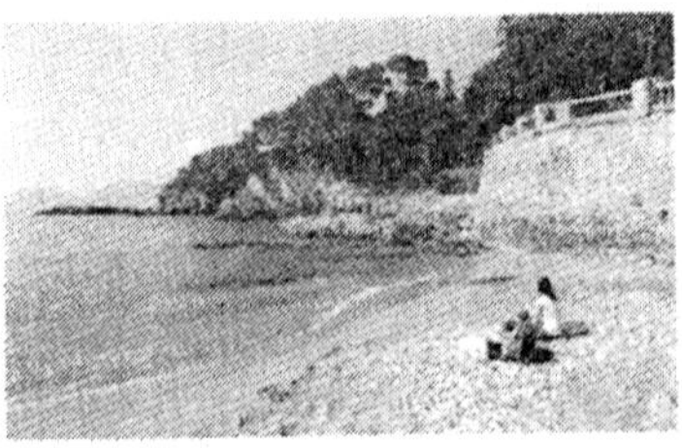

Social and Entertainment sectors: We must have a social life – making friends and meeting them and enjoying life with them. We must have relatives whom you love to meet and visit them for functions. This life often removes boredom from our life and make it enjoyable. To enjoy the social life longer remember one vital point – help your friend and avoid taking their help. This will make your social life better and better. Visiting theatres, going to picnics, travelling along with friends and relatives are lovely ways to share happiness.

Ego and Jealousy Sectors: These two are often seen making obstructions in our happy life and often be a constant source of our stresses. Ego is the tendency of people to show off their good characters and demand appreciation from others. True, everyone has some unique features and why not to show it off. Some people over do it and try to show faults of others so that others appear inferior to them. Other members of the family, friends and colleagues continuously feel stress from such people. The problem aggravates further if more people in the same group have ego problem. Then both of them do not tolerate each other and continuously produce stress for each other. To cut down ego, the golden rule is to develop the habit of agreeing to the opposite party that they are better than you. If you find it difficult to do this , search for your own faults and look for the good qualities of the other persons. It becomes easy to lead a stress free life if you learn to cut down ego.

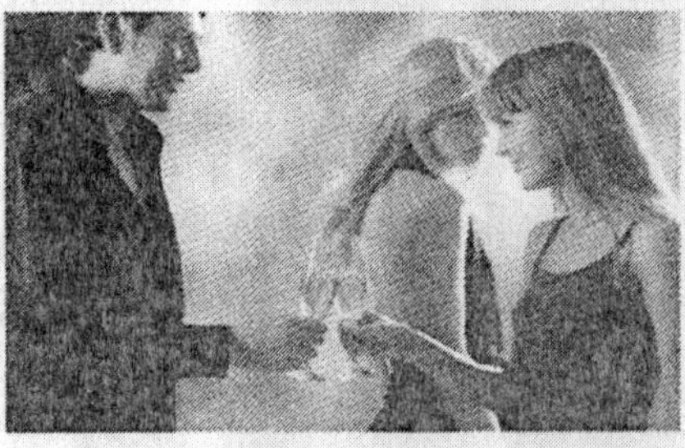

Jealousy is the habit of feeling bad when others succeed. It may be a family member, friend or a colleague or a neighbour who has done very well and you have a tendency to say " It's not a big deal." Remember in this world you are like a drop in the ocean. There are so many people who are better or worse than you in every aspect. Try to appreciate other's good habits, success and still feel good about it. Try to excel in life and feel happy.

Health: Ill health is a source of continuous stress. We do not usually feel it till we loose our health. If you have everything in life (money, name, fame, good family, love, social life) and the health is lost, then everything is lost. So take care of your health. Inculcate healthy habits(walking, exercise, meditation, relaxation),

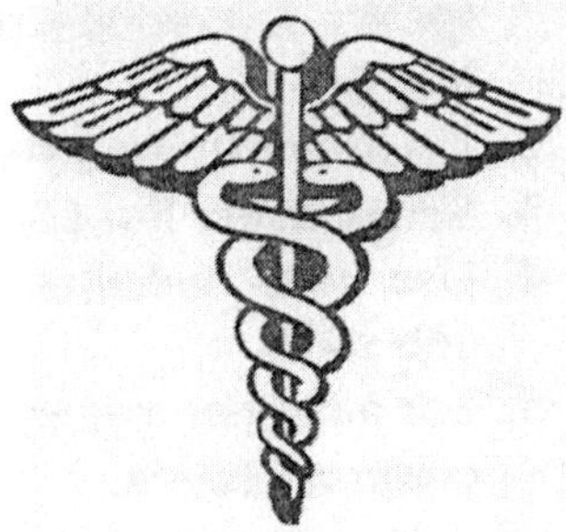

have healthy food and undergo regular medical check up to take care of your health.

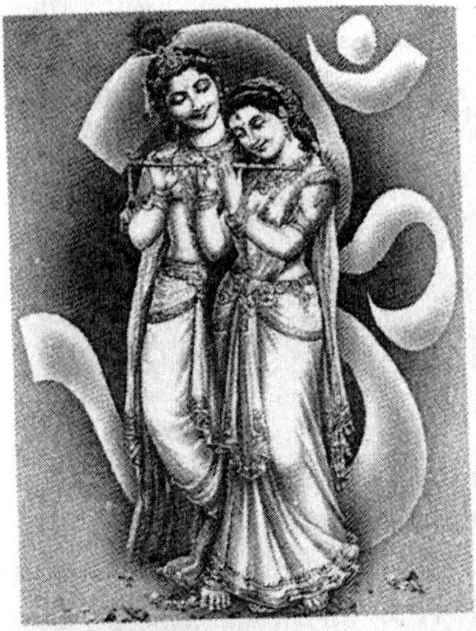

Spiritual sector: This is the sector of God. Even if you have achieved all the success in every sector of life – peace will not be there until you take shelter of God. Even the mighty, the powerful realize that they have to have faith in the almighty to get the real bliss. So develop faith in God, Allah, guru or any service to community that you feel will take you closer to God. Bliss will come to you. This sector is like vaccination against stress. You will become immune to small stresses of life if you develop your spiritual sector

9. COMMUNICATION SKILL

The art of talking or communication is very important for avoiding stress for an executive, official, teacher, professional, family man or woman. Half of our social stresses are due to bad communication skills. Some tips about this aspect are as follows :

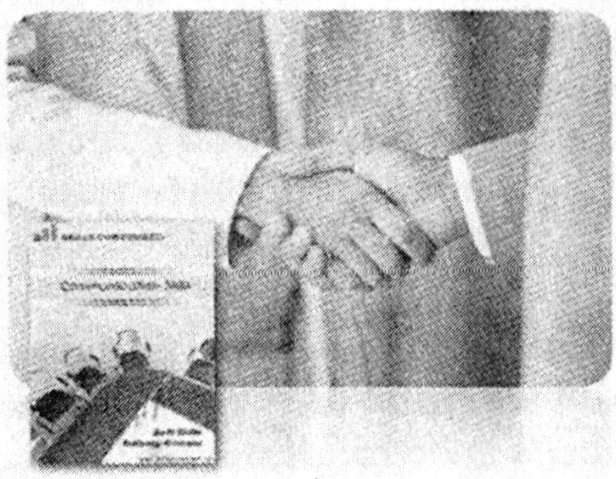

1. Listen when the other person speaks. Everyone wants to be heard.
2. Do not criticize directly. Don't insult. Only express your feeling.
3. Speak softly but come to the point.
4. Use your understanding of non-verbal communication before you start.
5. For a regular and smooth communication bring down the tone of communication.

Example:

	Good Communication	**Bad Communication**
Father to son	If you had done the job the way I said - his work would have been successfully completed.	You don't know how to work. You never do things properly. I know you will fail. You are useless.
Husband to wife	The pink sari will look better. Why don't you change this blue dress to pink?	You don't have any sense of dressing. This blue dress looks awful. When will you improve?

10. RELEASING AND MANAGING STRESS

Once we have produced stress – the sooner it can be managed and released –the better. Even with the best of efforts it is not possible to stop the production of stress completely. To manage stress and release stress the following tips may be useful.

Managing stress:

A. When you are angry:

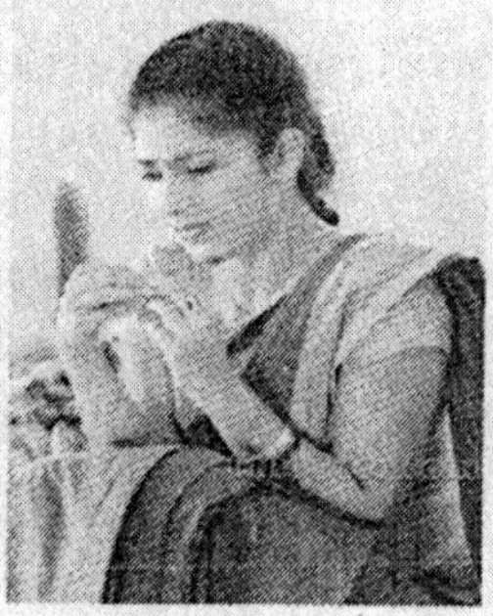

1. Do not act in haste. Let your anger simmer down.
2. Think of the positive side of criticism.
3. Use anger creatively - perform some job which needs your participation only e.g. clear a pending account work or read a tax chapter.
4. Talk to your close associate or friend.
5. Learn the art of forgiving.

B. When the anger has cooled down but a chronic stress is present:

1. Try to reach the root cause of the problem. Suggest an honest answer or solution.
2. Train yourself to understand non-verbal communication, half of what one talks gets reflected non-verbally.
3. Change your own dialogue, once you know you have been wrong.
4. Be persistent in small promises or your words.

5. Assertive social conversation - assert your need and do not suffer because of this.
6. Understand your critic.
7. Respond to your critic appropriately.
8. Make a workable compromise

C.Developing moral values (Anuvrat)

Erosion of moral values is one of the major causes of the social, cultural and behavioral decay in modern times. Everybody knows about this but somehow want to be unconcerned. For building a good personality we must follow the principles of Anuvrat which believe in the following:

1. Existence of others
2. Unity of mankind
3. Communal harmony
4. Non-violence
5. Limitation of acquisition and of consumption
6. Integrity in behaviour
7. Purity of means
8. Fearlessness and truthfulness.

D. Development of will power:

Will power is often the key behind a successful executive. Introspection during Preksha or Kayotsarg is one good tool for development of will power. Sticking to fairness and moral principles make a significant increment in the will power. Every person has unlimited will power, but it is never fully explored. Contemplation helps in this process immensely.

E. Contemplation :

A deep thought or repeated reinforcement of thoughts affects the Psycho-neuro-endocrine and Psycho-neuro-immune system to create changes in the body and mind. A headache can disappear, an enmity can turn into friendship and so on This procedure has immense power to solve chronic problems. A large number of practice procedures are available. With proper training the practice of contemplation improves gradually.

F. Jotting down Exercises :

Some chronic problems can be solved by simply jotting them down. We could then sketch the creation and solution to these problems. The remedies become very clear after such an exercise. Try to note down how many times you got stressed on a day. Write the occasions. Now try to solve each by different means as given by practical suggestions in the book. Using communication skills and adjustments of internal factors can solve many problems. Try some more choices. You can work wonders!

Releasing Stress:

The following points can be very useful for releasing stress:

a. Go to the temple, church or masjid. Perform puja or pray to God. Completely submit to Him.
b. Share your stress with someone. This is also called catharsis. This releases stress very quickly.
c. Sit and take sips of water from a glass. Take half an hour to finish and just do not do anything.
d. Start doing something that you like – like your hobby. It may be a music, a movie, game, reading magazine, listening to news.
e. Change the topic of discussion to something more interesting.
f. Doing Yoga ,meditation and Kayotsarg can also release the stress quickly.

11. YOGA FOR STRESS MANAGEMENT:

The following Yogic practices may be very vital techniques to release stress.

A. **Health rejuvenating exercises (HRE):** These are a set of movements to gear up your body and to develop co-ordination. They are for the preparation of the body. You should spend about 10 minutes on these movements everyday. These are Yoga based exercises to release stress.

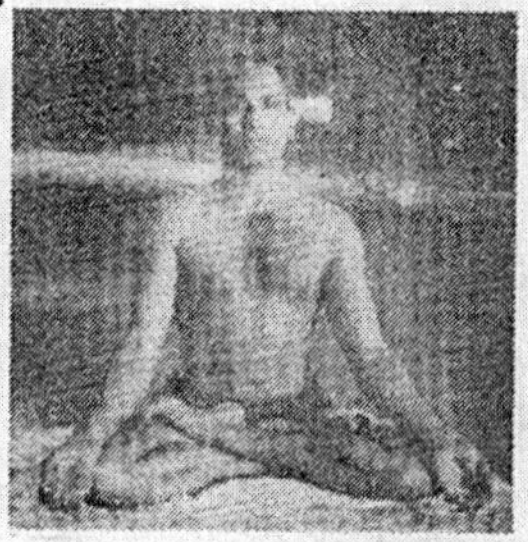

B. **Asanas or Yogic Postures :** These are for stretch and relaxation of the muscles and for increasing suppleness of the body. We advise you only six simple asanas which can be performed in 10 minutes.

C. **Pranayama:** Practice of Deep Breathing by alternate nose breathing (nadisodhan or Anulom Vilom Pranayama) is also a very good way to release stress.

D. Kayotsarg : This is a very effective method of relaxing your body and mind. This can be done for five minutes whenever you are tensed - whether it is at work or at home. You can do it for longer durations also.

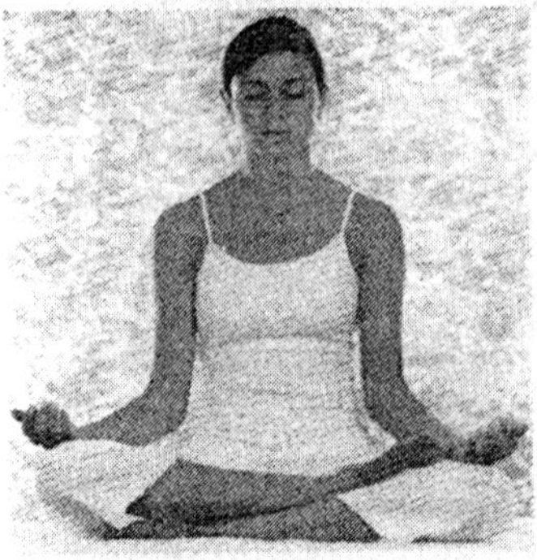

E. Preksha Meditation : Preksha means seeing deeply. It is a unique kind of meditation and is an extraordinary tool for relaxation. This meditation is one of the best ways to control the Emotional brain. Stress reduction is never complete unless the emotional brain is under control. The details will be dealt with later.

F. Contemplation : Contemplation is reinforcement of a positive idea by thought. Many problems can be solved by the practice of contemplation.

Time Management:

We have 24 hours in a day. Each one of us starting from the President of USA to the top most industrialist or a beggar are same in this regard. And all of them manage their work in the same time frame. How better you complete all your duties or responsibilities depends on your time management skills. You must plan. Best is to decide a long term plan and then from time to time sort out a small time schedule. For example, for the period you are on tour or preparing for an important meeting.

Sleep duration should ideally be of 6 to 7 hours. Keep atleast 1-2 hours for your family on a week day and try to spend maximum part of the holidays with the family. Daily chores should take about 2-3 hours (Bathing, dressing, breakfast etc.). Rest of your time is for work.

Now, set your priorities and divide your time. If you feel your duties are difficult to manage within a given time span, then consider delegating some duties to your junior or refuse the job. Try to stick to your daily routine and relax on holidays. If we analyze candidly, we will find that many of us do not actually spend our time working.

12. TIME MANAGEMENT

A list of Time Wasters is provided below :

1. Telephone interruptions
2. Meetings
3. Visitors
4. Socializing
5. Lack of information
6. Excessive Paper work
7. Communication breakdown
8. Lack of policies, procedures and coordination
9. Lack of competent personnel
10. Red tape
11. Procrastination
12. Failure to delegate
13. Unclear objectives
14. Failure to set priorities
15. Crisis management
16. Poor scheduling
17. Lack of self discipline
18. Attempting to do too much at one time
19. Lack of relevant skills.

Chapter-6

Yoga for High Blood Pressure Patients

INTRODUCTION

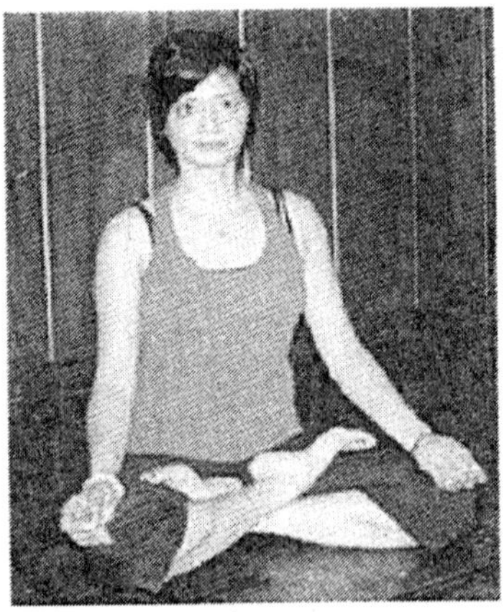

Yoga and relaxation have been successfully used for the amelioration of high blood-pressure and coronary heart disease over the past few decades. Recent researches have proved that this form of treatment not only reduces high blood-pressure but also reduces the serum cholesterol levels, serum triglyceride levels, serum free fatty acid, blood glucose, body weight and coronary artery disease. No form of medicine is as effective as yoga in the treatment of coronary heart disease. Unlike medical drugs, this form of therapy has no side effects. Yogic practice also improves physical fitness and helps to improve the individual's efficiency. Here, in this book, I am recommending a particular life-style enhancement intervention based on Preksha Yoga.

DEFINITION OF YOGA

Yoga is the philosophical doctrine(way of living) developed in India at about 500 BC based on moral principles, meditational techniques and a special type of physical training called Hatha Yoga which involves control of posture and respiration. It is said to bring about the right interaction, combination, co-ordination of the mind and body.

OTHER DEFINITIONS

Union between Prana (Vital Force) and Maha Shakti (Universal Energy)

Stopping of fluctuations or disturbances of consciousness (Chitta)

Achievement of inner equilibrium (Samatvam), harmony

Yoga is the skill of work.

EIGHT STEPS OF YOGA FROM PATANJALI

Yoga, one of the oldest sciences, is 5000 years old. It has been described in ancient literatures like the Veda and Agams. Rishi Patanjali, the Father of Yoga (300 BC) has been the most well known Yoga Guru. According to Patanjali there are 8 steps of Yoga, viz. Yam (यम), Niyama (नियम), Asana (आसन), Pranayama (प्राणायाम), Pratyahar (प्रत्याहार), Dharana (धारणा), Dhyana (ध्यान), Samadhi (समाधी).

Yama:	Restraints and controls : Non violence - (Ahimsa)		
	Truth	-	(Satya)
	Non stealing	-	(Astha)
	Celibacy & Self restraint-		(Bhramhacharya)
	Non hoarding	-	(Aparigraha)
Niyama:	Observations : Purity, cleanliness- (Saucha)		
	Satisfaction	-	(Santosh)
	Devotion to God	-	(Tapas)
	Self learning	-	(Swadhyay)
	Dedication	-	(Tyag)
Asana:	Physical Holds		
Pranayama:	Control of breathing		
Pratyahara:	Negation of hunger; control over senses		
Dharana:	Concentration; fixation of mind		
Dhyana:	Contemplation; flow of concentration.		

MEDITATION

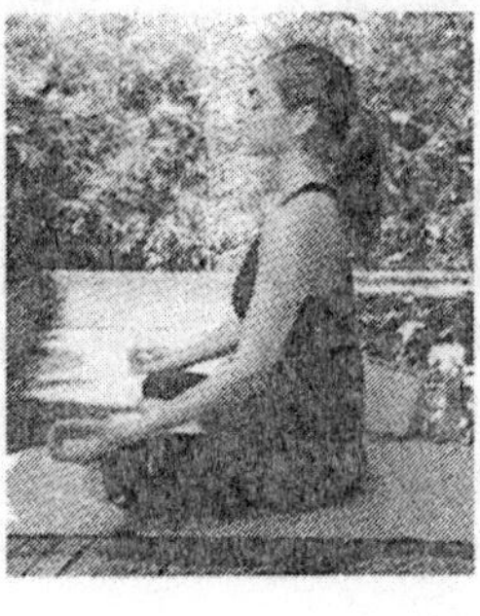

Meditation is the most important part of Yoga which helps in reducing high blood pressure. Stress comes from the mind or brain. Meditation relaxes the mind or brain. Through meditation we are also able to control our emotional mind. In majority of cases our rational mind understands the situations (external stresses) and adjusts itself. But our emotional mind – which controls our anger, greed, sorrow, revenge – plays havoc. Meditation is the single practice which helps in taming the emotional mind. Any real follower of Yoga (especially meditation) cannot become angry.

Scientifically speaking, there are four important components of meditation:

a. Quiet Atmosphere
b. Comfortable Posture
c. Passive Attitude
d. Follow the Theme

Meditation leads to relaxation by producing alpha waves in the brain. They also help to tame our Emotional brain so that we can control our emotions better.

Gist of doing meditation:

If you want to meditate first thing to assure is that the surroundings are non stimulating to the brain. All our sense organs must stop providing cues to the brain so that brain relaxes. For this you should make sure there is very little light in the place and you should close your eyes. For the sound disturbance – make sure that there is no one making any noise. That is why meditation is done early morning when the disturbance from sound is minimum. In meditation halls people are told to maintain silence. Now during meditation you should not touch anything (it stops the stimulation from skin), smell any stimulating odor (it stops stimulation from nose) or eat any thing (it stops signals from the tongue. This stops signals from all your five sense organs(Gyanendriyas). You should stop talking, try not to move any part of the body. This relaxes the brain.

The next thing to make sure is that any joint or muscle of the body does not give pain stimulus to the brain. For this your posture should be comfortable, you should not fall down even if the body is completely relaxed. Postures like Sukhasana are now most suitable for this purpose. Those who can not sit on the floor even chair or sofa can be used and the person should be comfortable. The spine should be preferably straight during meditation. This assures that the disturbance from the body is minimal to the brain.

The third part of the meditation is to stop the signals and chains of thoughts being generated from your brain. These thoughts that will come to your mind now are memories of past (Smriti in Hindi), problems of the present (Chintan in Hindi) and possibilities of future (Kalpana in Hindi). All these will keep on chaining up with more related topics in your mind and the whole lot of stresses will now generate in your brain. Try to stop these chains of thoughts. This is very difficult. But more you can do this – the better will be your relaxation.

The fourth part of meditation is concentrating your mind on a particular theme or object. It may be your breath, a mantra, moon, blue sky, statue of God or anything. You can also concentrate your mind to a thought (this is called Anupreksha). For the high BP patient it may be "my blood pressure is reducing, I am relaxing, my whole body is relaxing…". You can concentrate on some particular parts of the brain (these are called Chakras or centers in Yogic language). Keep doing this for five to ten minutes. This completes meditation. One thing you should remember – during meditation you should not sleep and should remain complete awake.

Themes of Meditation

Earth Elements	:	Black Dot, Statue of God
Water Elements	:	River, Lake, Sea
Sound Elements	:	Word, Mantra, Japa, Bhajan
Fire Elements	:	Lamp, Candle
Nature Elements	:	Blue Sky, Dense Forest, Sun, Moon, Ice-peaks, Sea
Body Elements	:	Sarir (Organs), Limbs, Breathing
Psychic Centres	:	Kundalini
Colours	:	Orange, Green, White
THOUGHTS	:	ANUPREKSHA

SCIENTIFIC EFFECTS OF YOGA AND MEDITATION ON THE BODY

Medical research has already proved the effects of Yoga, Asana, Meditation

1. Blood Pressure
2. Pulse rate or Heart rate
3. Catecholamines
4. Oxygen consumption
5. Positive conversion of patients with Type A personality to TypeB
6. Anxiety Level

7. Flexibility
8. Serum Cholesterol
9. Blood Glucose ê (control diabetes)
10. Smoking
11. Physical Fitness
12. Improves Sleeplessness
13. Better availability of oxygen in lungs
14. Reversal of Heart Disease

The Sub-groups of yoga

Yoga therapy for high Blood pressure would involve five different groups of practices

1. Health Rejuvenating Exercises (HRE)
2. Asanas or Relaxing Postures
3. Pranayama or Breathing exercises
4. Kayotsarg or Relaxation
5. Meditation: Preksha Dhyaan
6. Moral Teaching & Anupreksha

Training and Timings:

The total duration of the daily practice of yoga should be about 40 to 60 minutes. However, Meditation can be practiced for longer periods, if one desires. The best time to practice Yoga and Relaxation is early in the morning which is also very convenient for a regular practitioner or professional individual who has to go to work everyday. Ideally, the stomach should be empty during the practice. Some of the optimum requirements other than these are loose and comfortable fitting clothes, quiet surroundings and an adequately ventilated room.

The training will consist of four separate sessions each of 2 hours duration, where the patients along with their spouses will be taught all these procedures. They can however, consult the manual from time to time while they practice at home to verify any procedure.

RULES & REGULATIONS

1. **Regularity** and punctuality in practice is essential.
2. **The time** fixed for practice should be maintained. Early morning hours are best suited for such types of practices because the bowels are clean and the stomach is empty. For some people evening hours are also suitable. At least a 2 hour gap must be allowed between the taking of meals and practice.

3. **Food:** If one needs a cup of coffee or tea or milk can be taken half an hour before the practice of asanas, the ideal goal of the practitioner is to stop tea and coffee completely.
4. **Place:** Clean and airy place without noise or disturbance is ideal for doing exercises and Asanas.
5. **Dress:** Comfortable, loose and a light dress is good for such practices.
6. **Sleep:** About 6 to 8 hours sleep is required daily for an adult. If one goes to bed early, it will be possible to have sound sleep and to get up early in the morning. Then and only it becomes possible to maintain the proper timing for Yoga practice.
7. **Rest:** While doing Asanas if one feels tired, he/she should take rest. Never cross the limits of your capacity. Your capacity will increase slowly. After completion of the Asanas five minutes of Kayotsarg (muscular relaxation) is necessary. After that meditation can be practiced.

THE YOGIC DIET

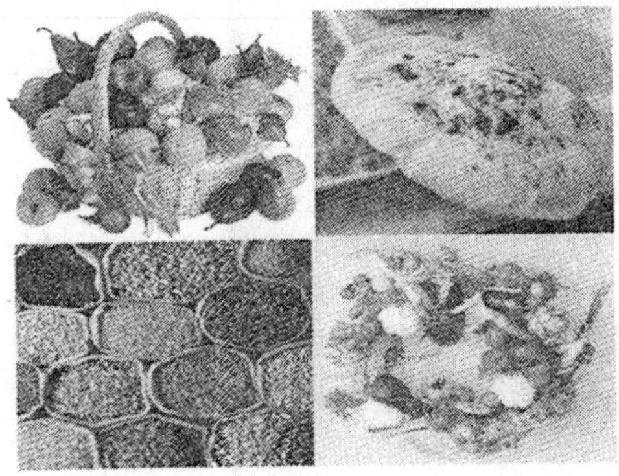

Under the Yogic system, diet is classified as **Satvik, Rajsik and Tamsik**. For people who have coronary heart diseases, the **Satvik system of diet** is best suited. The Satvik diet has all the cereals, dals, fruits and vegetables which are in very close association to nature. Although milk and yogurt are also a part of the Satvic food system, the **Saaol Heart Program** reduces their consumption to a minimal permissible amount which is essential for the reversal of the blockages in the coronary arteries, as we shall see later on. The diet should be fat-free and have no cholesterol, as far as possible. The intake of white sugar and salt should be moderate. Tea and coffee, or other caffeine containing beverages should be excluded from the diet.

The diet should have a considerable quantity of roughage. The covering (husks) of all grains, legumes, vegetables and fruits are fiber containing foods and also have some minerals, enzymes and antioxidants which are extremely essential for reducing the cholesterol level in the blood.

An ideal intake in a day should be as follows:

Breakfast: Fruits, a bowl of daliya made of oat-bran, whole wheat, maize, millets and sprouted grains.

Lunch: Roti preferably made of whole wheat, gram and soya flour, vegetable salads, dal, chatni, rice and soups. Atta 50% wheat, 25% Soya and 25% bengal gram.

Afternoon: Fruits and herbal tea.

Dinner: Dalia, khichari, kari, boiled leafy vegetables, sprouted and steamed grams like chick-peas (Bengal gram), moong, beans etc. Chapaties can also be taken.

HEALTH REJUVENATING EXERCISES

These few postural movements mentioned below are preparatory before beginning the next step i.e. Asanas. They are to be practised before beginning the Yogic training.

They are:-

I. For the Eyes
II. For the Neck
III. For the Ears
IV. For the Face
V. For the Shoulders
VI. For the Chest
VII. For the Waist
VIII. For the Thighs
IX. For the Knees
X. For the Ankle Joints
XI. For the Toes & Heels

I. For The eyes

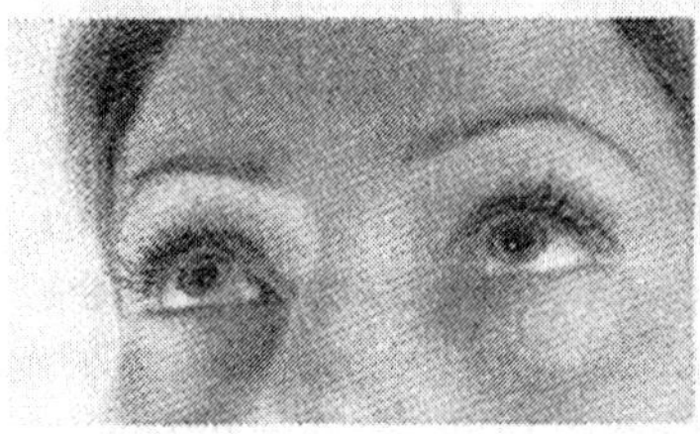

A) *Position:*

Stand at ease.

B) *Movements:*

1. Keeping the head fixed look up and down a few times.
2. Then look to your right and left, and further rotate your eyeballs. Try to cover the maximum range of vision.
3. Put your palms over both eyes after warming and blink a few times.

II. For the NECK

A) ***Position*:**

Stand at ease.

B) ***Movements*:**

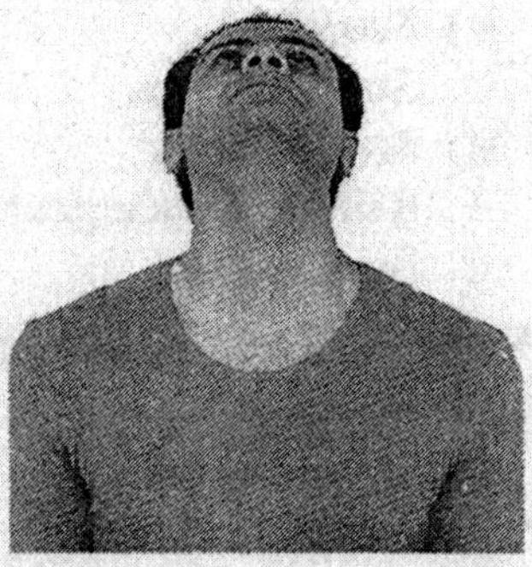

1. Rub the hands together vigorously for 10 counts. Rub the back portion of the neck alternatively.
2. Repeat the same from the front side five times.
3. Bend your neck backward as far as possible and then touch your chin on the chest by bending forwards. Repeat this procedure five times.
4. Turn your neck thoroughly from the left side, over the shoulders and vice-versa.
5. Bend your neck alternatively to both sides, try to touch the ears to the left and right shoulders alternately.
6. Rotate the neck starting with the chin, touching the chest with the eyes closed, turn to the right with the eyes opened, ears touching the shoulders and further through the back looking up and left ear touching the left shoulder and back to chin with eyes closed. Do it on the other side also (2 rounds).

III. FOR THE EARS

A) Position:

As above. Hold upper portion of both ears with thumb and index fingers.

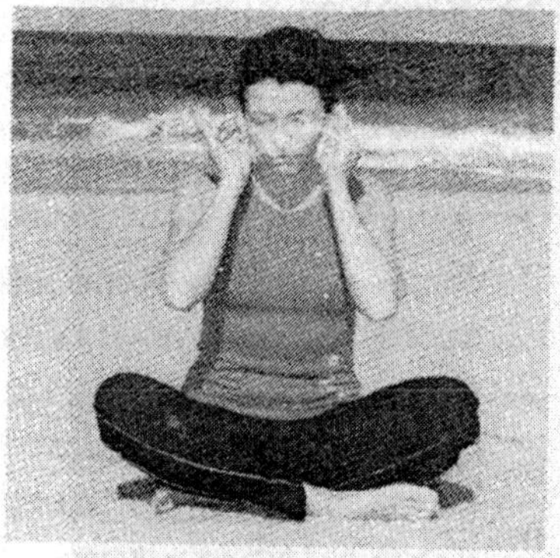

B) ***Movement:***

1. Pull up both ears.
2. Pull straight out the middle portion
3. Pull down the lower lobes.
4. Cover both the ears completely with the palms, press and relax without taking away the hands to create vacuum in the ears.
5. Make fist with three fingers and thumb, leaving the index free. Now with the index fingers rub the front of the ears.
6. With the same fingers now rub the back side of the ears.

IV. FOR THE FACE

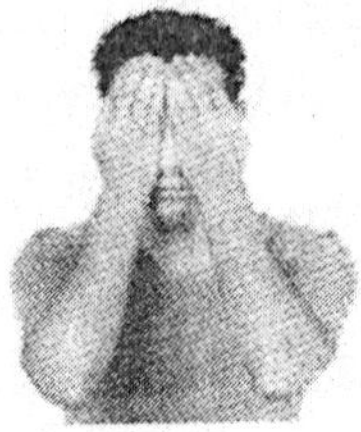

A) ***Position:***

Stand at ease.

B) ***Movements:***

1. Rub your face gently using both the palms.
2. Feel relaxed.

V. FOR THE SHOULDERS

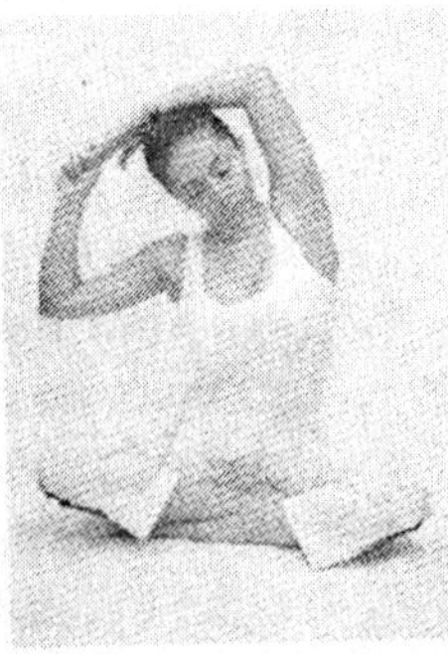

A) ***Position:***

Stand at ease.

B) ***Movement:***

1. Keep your arms hanging straight down by your sides with fists closed. Raise the shoulders up, while inhaling and bring down while exhaling, without bending the elbows.
2. Rotate the shoulders from back to front keeping the arms relaxed and repeat it from front to back also (five time each).
3. Bend your arms, fingers and thumb together touching the shoulders. Inhale and rotate the arms from forward to backward and then from back to front.

VI. FOR THE CHEST

A) ***Position:***

Bend both arms inwards, bringing the palms over the chest, facing it, with middle fingers meeting at the middle of the sternum.

B) ***Movement:***

1. Inhale and extend the left hand, exhale and bring the hand to its former position. Repeat the exercise with the right hand (five times each) and then do it with both the arms five times.
2. Keep the hand in front on the thighs. Inhale and raise the left arm touching the ear without bending, bring the arms down and exhale. Repeat it with right arm and then with both the arms five times.

VII. FOR THE WAIST

A) ***Position:***

Keep the feet apart as per the shoulders width, arms should be hanging down by the sides of the body.

B) ***Movement:***

1. Raise hands while inhaling, bend at the waist about 30° or more to

the left while exhaling, bring the left hand near the knee, bend the neck to the left, drop the left hand also over the head inhale and exhale for 3 times. Reverse the process and come to the normal posture. Repeat this on the right side (2 rounds).

2. Lock the fingers and raise hands.
   (a) Turn palms upwards towards the sky.
   (b) Bend at waist 30° or more to the left, arms straight with ears towards the left.
   (c) Return to the position (1)
   (d) Bring the arms down, repeat it to the right (2 rounds)
3. Keep the palms together.
   (a) Inhale and raise the hands upwards, arms straight touching the ears.
   (b) Exhale and bend 30° or more to the left. (Inhale & exhale for 5 times)
   (c) Return to position (a).
   (d) Bring the arms down, repeat it to the right.
4. (a) Inhale, raise the arms to the shoulder level, chest width apart, keeping the palms facing each other.
   (b) Twist at the waist so that the right hand goes to the left shoulder and the left hand goes to the right hip. (Inhale and exhale 5 times).
   (c) Inhale and come to position (a).
   (d) Exhale and bring the hands down repeat the same on the right side (3 rounds)

VIII. FOR THE THIGHS & HIPS

A) ***Position:***

Stand straight, keep the legs apart about 15 to 20 cm.

B) ***Movement:***

Strike the buttocks with the heel; alternately.

IX. FOR the KNEES

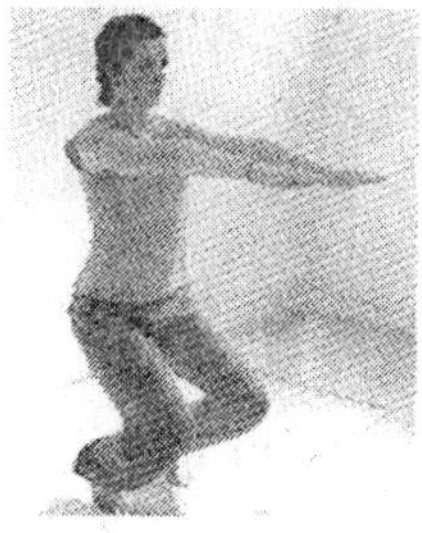

A) ***Position:***

Keep the above standing position.

B) ***Movement:***

1. Let your left heel hit the hip; then stretch forward feeling jerk at knee. Do it with right leg also. Repeat it five times.

2. Place your hands on the waist keeping your thumbs in the front. Keep both feet 30 cms apart. Keep the body straight and bend knees as low as possible, then, come up. Repeat this 5 times.

X. FOR the ANKLE JOINTS

Raise the left leg a little above the ground. Move the ankle upward and downward 5 times. Then rotate from the ankle clockwise and anti-clockwise. Repeat it with the right leg also.

XI. FOR THE TOES & HEELS

Walk forwards on your toes, then walk backwards on your heels.

YOGA ASANA FOR LOWERING HIGH BP:

(A) STANDING POSTURES

1. Tadasana

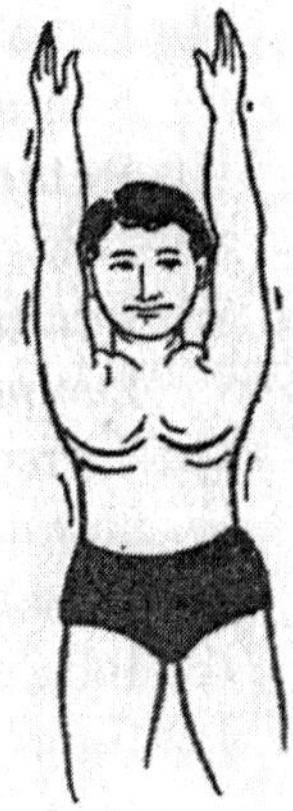

Position: Keeping both heels and toes parallel and 10 cm apart; arms by the side.

Movement: Inhale. Raise the arms up expanding the chest and abdomen slowly. Put the back side of the palms together, raise the body on the toes. Hold the posture looking at a point at eye-level. Keep the knees straight, bring the heels and arms down while exhaling as in the starting position.

Caution: Persons with slipped disc should not do this posture.

2. Padahastasana

Position: Stand erect with both feet together.

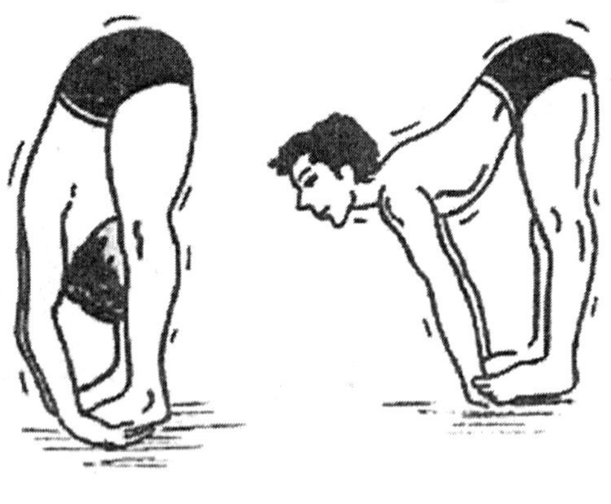

Movement: Raise the arms, palms facing forward over the head while inhaling. Exhale slowly while you bend forward, bring the palms down to hold the ankles and touch forehead to the knees. Try to keep the knees and ankles straight. While you bend your body up to the level where you can bend easily keep in mind that the goal is to touch the forehead to the knees. Slowly raise your body while inhaling and taking the arms up exhale and bring the arms down.

Caution: *The persons who have slipped disc (disc prolapse) should not do this asana.*

(B) SITTING POSTURES

3. Vajrasana

Position: Kneel down.

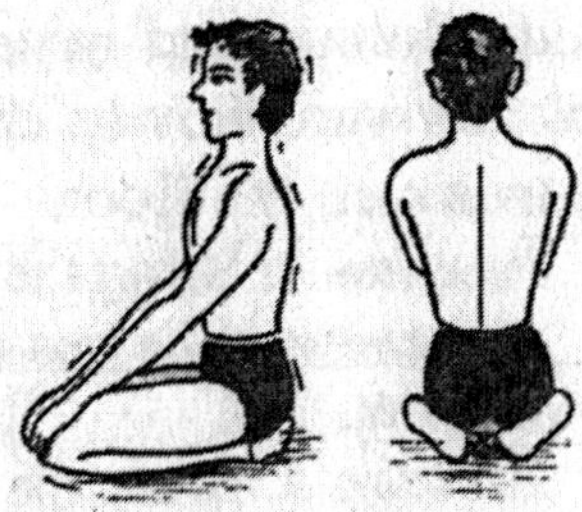

Movement: Assume kneeling position, heels open apart and toes together, soles upward. Sit on the soles, keeping the knees together. Inhale and exhale slowly and rhythmically.

4. Shasanksana

Position: Sit in Vajrasana, put palms together on the knees, keeping both arms straight.

Movement: Inhale and raise the joined arms over the head and arms should touch the ears. Exhale and bend forward touching, the floor with the palms. Inhale-Exhale and maintain this posture for five breaths. Inhale and raise the arms along with the head. Exhale and bring the hands down. Do it twice.

5. Pranayama (Nadi Shodhan Pranayama)

Sit in a comfortable posture and breathe normally. Close your right nostril with your thumb and inhale slowly through the left nostril. When the inhalation is complete, close the left nostril also and hold your breath for 2-3 seconds. Now lift the thumb from the right nostril and slowly exhale keeping the left nostril closed. Repeat the process by inhaling through the left nostril and exhaling through the right nostril. This is one cycle of Nadi-shodhan pranayama. Repeat this for 10 cycles.

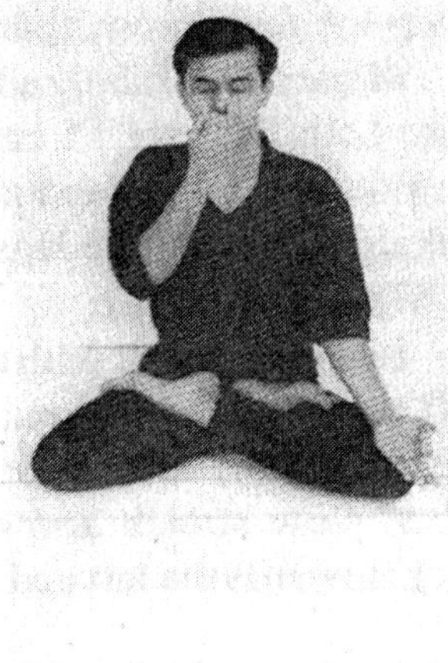

(C) LYING DOWN ON CHEST POSTURES

6. Modified Bhujangasana

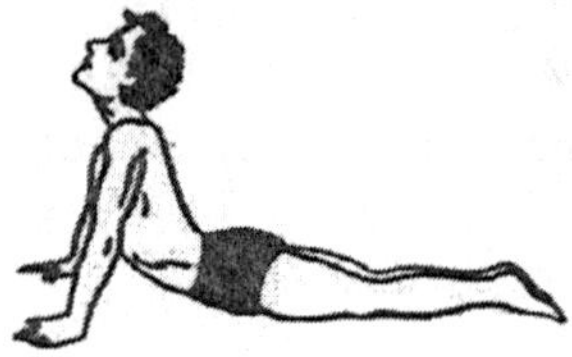

Position 1: Lie face down keeping heels and toes together. Place palms about 30 cm apart from the body.

Movement: Inhale and come up 15 cms. Exhale with hissing sound from the mouth, pulling the navel inside. Inhale and raise trunk on the palms and the thighs and look skyward slowly, exhale with hissing sound and bring down the trunk on the floor.

Position 2: Bring the hands near to the body by about 15 cms.

Movement: The rest of the movements are the same as that of the 1st position.

Position 3: Bring the hands near the body.

Movement: Inhale and raise the body 15 cm high from the floor. Exhale with hissing sound from the mouth. Inhale and raise the trunk a little more higher while the navel should touch the floor. Exhale with hissing sound and bring down the trunk on the floor. Spread hands beyond head on the right side of the face, keeping the toes together and heels open relax whole body. Turn the face and relax.

(d) LYING ON THE BACK ASANAS

7. Uattanpadasana

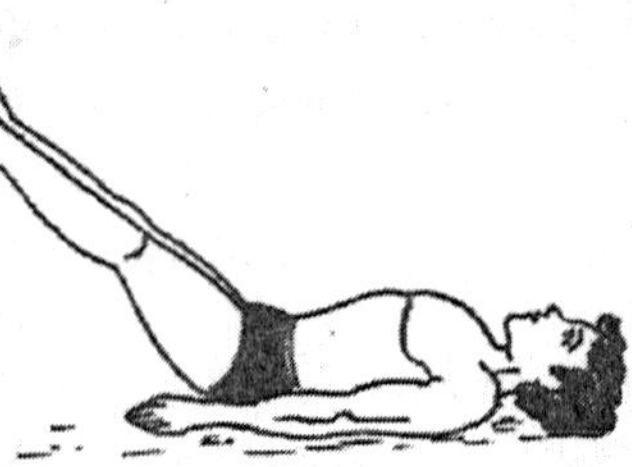

Position: Lie down on the back keeping the fingers locked together, under your neck, elbows on the ground. Keep the feet 15 cm apart.

Movement: Inhale and exhale and raise both the legs 15 cm high above the floor. Inhale and exhale for 5 times (inhale and bring the legs down and then exhale).

8. Merudandasan

Lie on the back with the arms stretched at right angles to the trunk. Lift the left heel and put it on the right foot in the space between the big toe and the second toe, thus, keeping the feet straight one above the other. Now stretch and rotate the upper part of the body (head and neck) towards the left and the lower parts (waist, thighs and feet) towards the right while you inhale. The left toe should now touch the ground and the arms and shoulders remain in the same position as before. Now come back to the original position while you exhale. Now repeat the same on the other side.

Repeat the whole process after changing the leg position (Right heel over the left foot).

Some more yoga asanas which are good for hypertension are:

9. Matsyasana

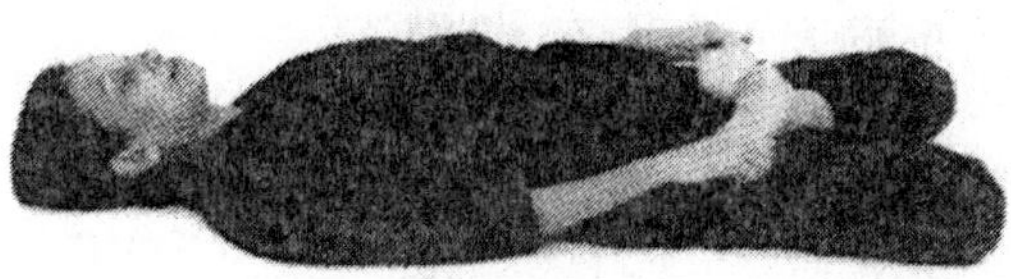

Sit in the lotus posture. Lie down on the back raise the trunk with the help of elbows and head (on the ground). Hold both the toes with the hands. Let the arched trunk rest on the head and buttocks.

10. Ardha-Matsyasana

Those who are unable to perform the Matsyasana, can practice this asana. Instead of assuming the lotus posture, spread the legs and with help of the elbows raise the body up and bend the neck backword; touch the head on the ground and the hands on the thighs. With the help of the elbows make the head straight and relax.

KAYOTSARGA

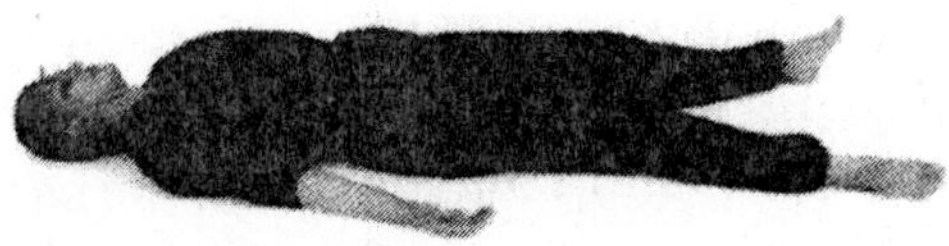

The first step of meditation is Kayotsarga. This is relaxation with self-awareness. Keep your body steady, relaxed and free from tension. Keep your spine and neck straight but without stiffness. Relax all the muscles of your body. Let your body become limp.

Practice steadiness of body at least for five minutes. Keep your body completely steady, as motionless as a statue. Do not allow the limbs of your body to move. No movement at all.

Kayotsarga has two implications—complete relaxation of the body and self-awareness. For achieving complete relaxation of the body, mentally divide it into several parts and concentrate your mind on each part of the body one by one, from feet to head. Allow your mind to spread in the whole part—allow it to undertake a trip in the whole part; use the technique of auto-suggestion to relax the whole part and experience the resulting relaxation. Experience that each and every muscle, each and every nerve has become relaxed. And in the same way attain, the relaxation of the whole body. Use deep concentration and remain completely alert.

Detailed Instructions for Kayotsarg :

Starting with the big toe of your right foot, concentrate your mind on it. Allow your mind to spread throughout the big toe. Suggest the muscles and nerves to relax. Relax..... Relax..... Relax.....Experience their relaxation. Experience that they have become relaxed. In the same way, attain relaxation of the other parts of the right limb—the other toes, sole, heel, ankle, upper part of the foot, calf-muscles, knee, thigh, upto the hip-joint. In the same way relax the left limb upto the hip-joint.

Now achieve the relaxation of the middle portion of the body from the waist upto the neck. Concentrate your mind on each part one by one starting with the lower abdomen, relax the front, the back, the right side, the left side, the outside and the inside of your lower abdomen. Similarly relax the upper abdomen— the front, the back, the right side, the left side, the outside and the inside of your upper abdomen. Now through your navel enter the abdominal cavity and relax the large intestine, the small intestine, the kidneys, the spleen, the liver, the pancreas, the stomach and the diaphragm. Use auto-suggestion and achieve relaxation. Then concentrate your mind on the chest and relax the entire rib-cage. Beginning with the lowest rib, relax each and every rib in turn. Relax the front ribs, the back ribs, the right ribs and the left ribs. Now enter the chest and relax the right lung, the left lung and the heart by auto-suggestion. (Those who have got any heart trouble should pause here for a few minutes and by auto–suggestion slow down the heart to remove stress.)

Now achieve the relaxation of the neck muscles in the front and in the back. Then concentrate your mind on both the hands and arms one by one; starting from the thumb, relax the fingers, the palm, the wrist, the lower arm, the elbow, the upper arm and the shoulder. Experience that the whole of the middle portion of your body has become completely relaxed.

Now achieve the relaxation of the upper portion of body from throat upto the head. Here we have come to a bit more difficult part of the exercise. So far you were relaxing large muscles which respond quickly to your suggestion. But now we have to relax a large number of small and tiny muscles which are difficult to relax. First unclench your teeth and unlock your jaws and let your tongue go limp. Keep your lips softly closed. Now relax all the facial muscles; beginning with the chin, relax the lips, the inner portion of the mouth including the teeth, the gums, the palate and the tongue; then relax the cheeks, the nose, the ears and the temples, both the eyes, the forehead and the scalp, through auto-suggestion. Experience that the whole of your upper portion of the body has become completely relaxed.

Again allow your mind to travel from the head upto the feet and from the feet upto the head; this time rather quickly and check that there is no tension anywhere in the body. Experience that the whole body from the feet upto the head has become completely relaxed. Maintain the posture of Kayotsarga throughout the meditation session. Try to keep your body completely steady and motionless.

Now practice inner silence at least for five minutes through relaxation of the vocal cords (voice box). Concentrate your mind on the voice box inside the throat and completely relax it. Observe complete inner silence. There should be no vibrations in the voice box

PREKSHA MEDITATION

This system of meditation is based on the wisdom of ancient philosophy and modern scientific concepts. Meditation does not mean suppression of mental functions. The main aim of Preksha Dhyana is to purify the mental state. When the mind is clean, peace of mind automatically surfaces. Balance of mind, equanimity and the state of well being are experienced simultaneously.

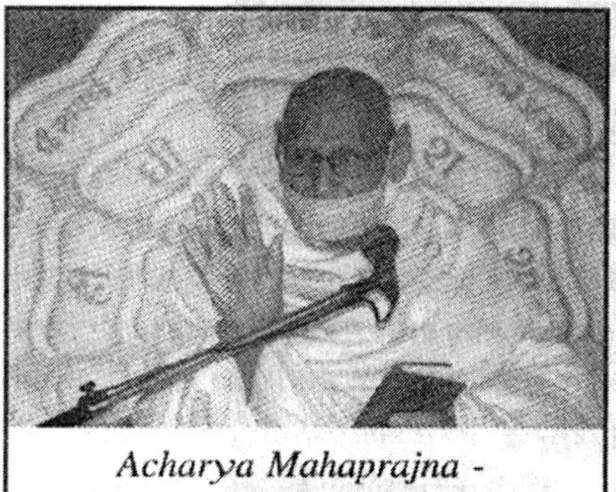

Acharya Mahaprajna - founder Preksha System

Preksha means "*Perception*" and **Dhyana** (Meditation) means "*Concentration*". So Preksha Dhyana means concentration of perception and not of thought. Mind is an instrument of thinking as well as perception. Perception is strictly concerned with the phenomena of the present. It is neither a memory of the past nor an imagination of the future. Perception of the present happenings must be a reality. In Preksha Dhyana, perception always means experiencing the benefits of the qualities of likes and dislikes. In due course of time our conscious mind becomes sharpened to perceive internal realities. There are steps of perception. To start with, perception of breath is an important element of this system.

The Technique:

Perception of Deep Breathing: Breathing is linked with the conscious mind. The mind is ever restless, it is extremely difficult to steady the wandering mind directly. An efficient and easy way to control mental activities is concentrated perception of breath, at the same time the rate of breathing is reduced from 15 to 17 per minute to 10 to 12 per minute and by further practice to 4 to 6 per minute.

***Step*: 1**

Do Kayotsarga, relax the whole body and feel it relaxed.

***Step*: 2**

Direct full attention to your breath, excluding all thoughts and sensations. Regulate your breathing, make it slow, deep and rhythmic. Focus your attention on the navel and become fully aware of contraction and expansion of the abdomen accompanying exhalation and inhalation simultaneously.

***Step*: 3**

Continuing the slow, deep and rhythmic breathing, shift your attention from the navel and focus it inside the junction of the nostrils, develop your attention on the process of respiration. Each and every inhalation and exhalation is perceived i.e. each and every breath is to be watched, felt and knowingly inhaled and exhaled.

***Step*: 4**

If distraction does occur, return your attention to your breathing. If it is frequent, then hold your breath for a few seconds and then breathe again normally.

Step: **5**

To finish the meditation, take two or three long breaths. Mahasprana for three times or sutras and pay obeisance by bending forwards.

ANUPREKSHA & MORAL CODE

Anupreksha means contemplation or reflection or thoughtful consideration. It can be used to get rid of many stressful aspects of our daily behavior. The urges, impulses, emotions, passions can be controlled by it. It also teaches us moral code. Our total life-style can be changed to a more relaxed, stressless and purposeful existence.

For heart patients, Anupreksha helps to open the blocked arteries. This practice of positive thinking has recently achieved validation from medical science, and this latest branch of medical science is called Psycho-neuro Immunology (PNI). According to PNI, whenever positive thinking is done, positive neuro-chemicals are released in the body fulfilling our requirements or wishes. Dr. Dean Ornish had also used this procedure in his life-style heart trial for opening the coronary arteries.

❑

Chapter-7

Habits to Change

For controlling blood pressure the following habits have to be changed and these are:

1. Stop smoking or consumption of Tobacco
2. Avoid stimulating drinks like tea and coffee
3. Sleep properly and adequately
4. Avoid alcohol
5. Read food labels
6. Increase physical activity during work or in daily life

Stop smoking and Tobacco:

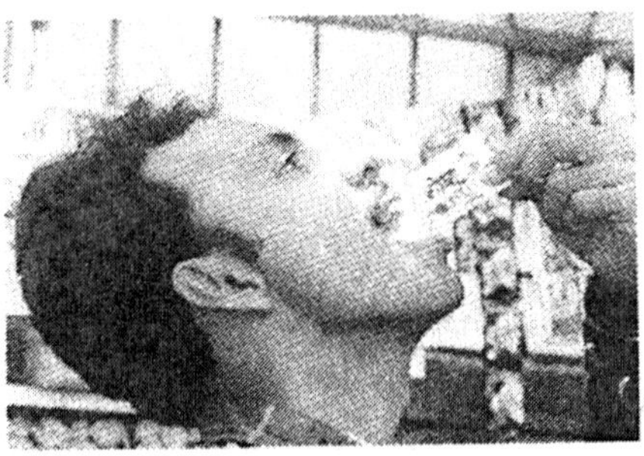

Smoking cigarettes, bidi, cigars are a must if you want to control high BP. Tobacco consumption of any kind – Zarda, khaini, gudaku, kimam, gutka, naswar are some of the forms of tobacco intakes in different parts of India. These are to be avoided completely. These tobacco products are not only bad for heart diaesase, cancer but also lead to spasm of the arteries and increase the Blood pressure.

Caffeine and tea are also to be avoided:

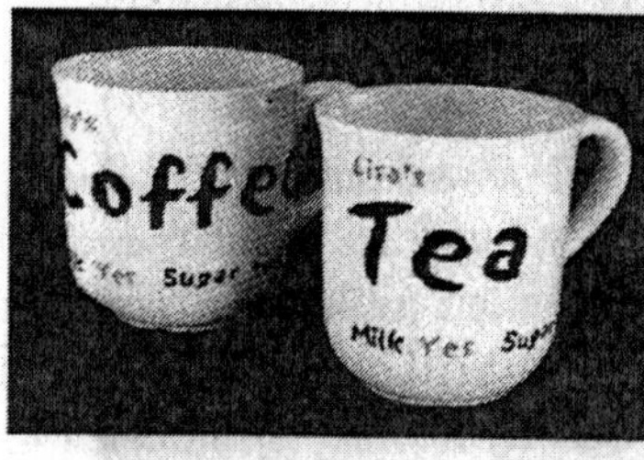

Tea and coffee are also stimulants to the brain. You must have observed that when you feel sleepy – a cup of tea or coffee can immediately wake you up by stimulating the brain. While on a long drive , when the driver feels sleepy – you stop the car in the road side restaurant so that he can have some strong tea or coffee. These products have Caffeine and nicotine which have the capacity of exciting the brain. It is better to replace tea and coffee with herbal drink, juice and soup. If you are very keen on drinking these stimulating drinks – look for decaffeinated drinks.

Have proper and adequate sleep:

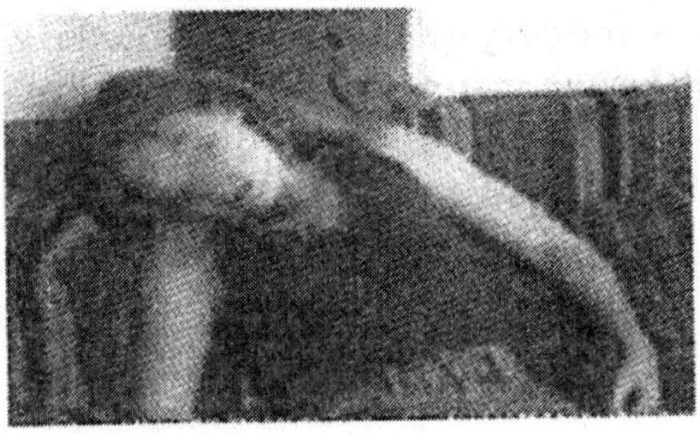

Our body and mind cannot work day and night. It needs rest and sleep is the best kind of rest. Sleep deprivation increases blood pressure. In today's life people are very busy and many do not find time to sleep adequately. Any adult after the age of 18 needs about 6-8 hours of sleep. After 50 years it can be 5-7 hours. Some people have time to sleep but stress and anxiety do not allow them to sleep. They must cut down the stresses by training of the mind and taming of the emotions. Yoga and meditation will also help. If there is tremendous stress – I would even recommend a sleeping pill for some time till the stress is solved.

Avoid alcohol

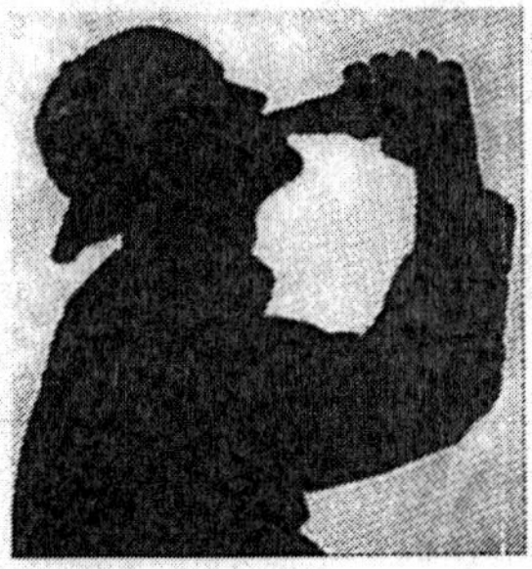

Alcohol does not go well with a relaxed mind and a healthy body. Small dosage of alcohol stimulate the brain and larger dosage inhibit the brain. Both are bad. It is addictive, leads to family stress, spoils nervous system, and not at all a good way to relax. Along with alcohol people usually consume high salt high fat foods. Patients of high blood pressure will be better off without alcohol.

Read food labels

Nowadays, food labels are compulsory with every packed food. They have to write the contents on the packet. Whenever you buy a food item make sure you observe for fats, salt content, calorie content, cholesterol content, caffeine and nicotine content. This habit will help you buy healthy and better food for your health and high blood pressure.

Increase Physical activity in daily life:

Drops of water can make the ocean. In our daily life we should imbibe more physical activity. Not using lift for going up till three floors or going down the stairs for any number of floors, picking up your glass of water, walking small distances which you would have gone by car, cleaning your own car, gardening, ironing your own clothes, arranging your books/room are some of the examples of physical activity in daily life. These add up to control your weight, making you stress free and reduce your cholesterol.

❑

Chapter-8

Walking and Exercises for High BP Patients

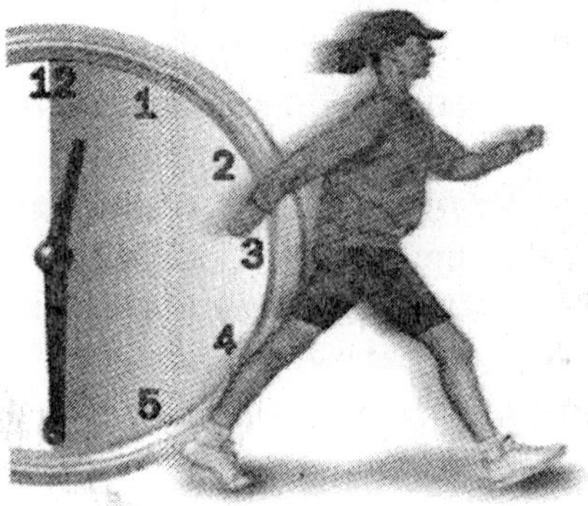

A minimum of thirty five minutes of walking is ideal for people with high BP and helps to reduce the Blood Pressure. This should ideally be done in the morning, but can be done at any time of the day. The speed of the walking should be according to your fitness. Walking with high exertion can increase the BP and a slow walk does not give any benefit. For a practical approach the walking should be in a speed where you cannot talk comfortably while walking. This speed can be called Sub-maximal speed.

Walking should be with a period of warm up (slow speed walk for the first few minutes) and end with gradual slowing down period (cooling down). It is ideal that there should not be lot of stops within this period of walk. Very commonly there will be breaks in walking because of busy schedule or travelling. It is better to walk where ever you are travelling.However, if there are breaks, walking should gradually be increased in speed and time to 35 minutes at submaximal speed.

Other types of low exertion physical exercise like aerobics, dancing, playing table tennis, cycling are also very good for high blood pressure patients. These exercises are called isotonic exercises. High strain exercises like Gym, lifting heavy weight, snooker, pushing exercises, wrestling are not suitable for high BP patients and should be avoided.

The following are the benefits of regular walking and exercises:

Physical Benefits

1. Enhancement of physical performance (ability to perform physical work without fatigue or strain on the heart)
2. Better control of Angina
3. Better control of Blood Pressure
4. Decreased susceptibility to Rhythm disturbances
5. Better control of Body Weight
6. Improvement of fat distribution
7. Greater efficiency of lung
8. Better Organ and limb circulation
9. Prevention of age related weakening of bones
10. Better cold and heat tolerance
11. Protection of the Joints
12. Decreased tendency to have hyperacidity
13. Better bowel function
14. Improved function and appearance of skin
15. Regression of Coronary Artery Blockage
16. Reduction in rate of recurrence of Heart Attacks
17. Increase in lifespan.

Biochemical Benefits

1. Reduction of low density Cholesterol (bad cholesterol)
2. Increase in High density (good) cholesterol
3. Reduction in Blood Triglyceride (Fat) levels
4. Better control of Diabetes Mellitus
5. Decreased tendency for spontaneous clots
6. Decrease in stress induced inappropriate hormone secretions.

Psychological Benefits

1. Enhanced energy, enthusiasm and self image
2. Decreased anxiety and depression
3. Better ability to cope with stress
4. Better relaxation and sleep
5. Less dependence on sleeping pills and drugs to control anxiety

Socio-Economic Benefits

1. Early return to gainful employment
2. Reduction in recurrent medical expenses.

Chapter-9

Medicines for Treatment of High Blood Pressure

- Introduction
- Advantages of Allopathic Medicines for High BP
- Monitoring of your BP during treatment
- Blood group of BP medicines
- Side effects
- Some more points

INTRODUCTION

As high blood pressure does not give any symptoms to a patient it is very common for high BP patients to avoid all medicines and even if they take medicines they take them irregularly. They even have worries and inhibitions about checking their Blood pressure and try to postpone the BP check up. This is not a good trend. This is more damaging in the long run.

Another problem is reluctance to start the medicines. Since it is a chronic disease – people are aware that the medicines will carry on for a long term or even may be life long. So, they try to avoid starting of BP medicines for years together even though they know that the disease is there and they are only postponing.

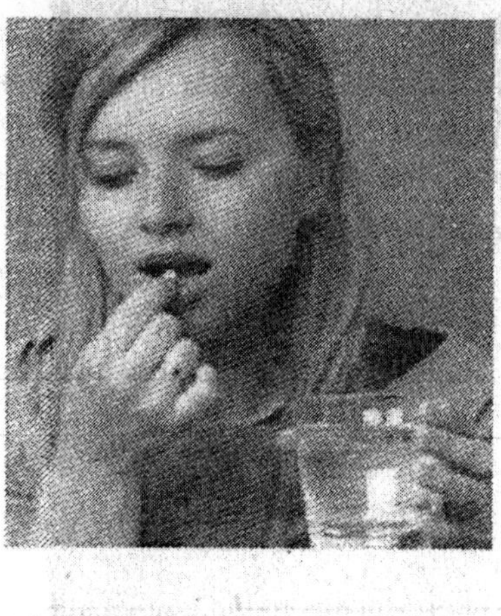

The doctors who they visit for general check up are mostly general physicians (called GPs) – mostly take High BP very lightly and to please the patient(or remain friendly) tell them “BP is slightly high, don’t worry”. Many of the GPs still have an idea that a BP of 140/90mmHg is normal after a certain age, which is not true (now a days the Best BP is 110/75 or 120/80 for any age). This happens because most of the GPs do not study the latest developments of medical science and stick to the information they had 20-30 years back.

One thing I must assure to a High blood pressure patient is that the medicines need not be taken lifelong and can be withdrawn if you can change your lifestyle, food, exercise and food pattern. Yoga and meditation is also tremendously useful. If you are overweight – reducing weight will also be extremely useful. I have got thousands of patients who have reduced their BP medicines substantially and stopped them completely as their BP returned to normal with lifestyle changes.

So, the general advice is if you have a BP which is continuously above 140/90 and you have not been able to control them with your efforts – please visit a physician and start (allopathic) the medicines advised by them. Keep taking the medicines regularly and keep checking your BP weekly. Go for a readjustment of these medicines if you find them higher than 120/80 figure. In the meantime start all the lifestyle advice that I have written for you and wait for the results. I promise, if you have been sincere to yourself, the results will be 100% there. You will be able to reduce medicines and may go completely off any medicines.

ADVANTAGES OF ALLOPATHIC MEDICINES FOR HIGH BP:

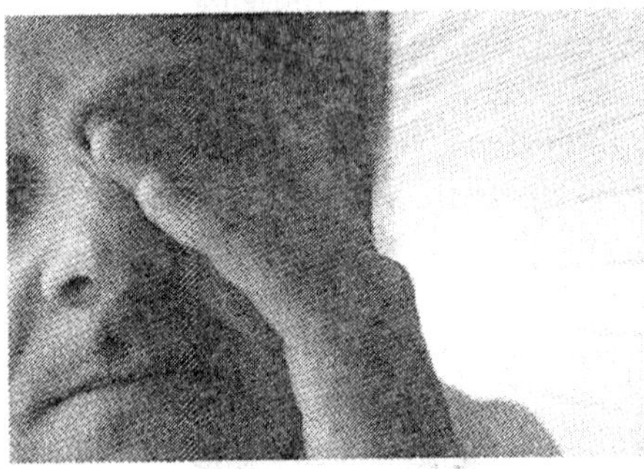

There is no doubt that most of the allopathic medicines are chemicals in nature and are not the best things for the body. But they have certain advantages. Lets list them:

1. They work for everyone and at every time.
2. They have been studied (researched) and tried on animals first, to prove their effects and side effects.
3. We know their mechanism of action.

4. Their dosages can be adjusted as and when required.
5. They work for a fixed time – 8 hours or 12 hours or 24 hours. So if taken at that interval they will be able to reduce your BP for 24 hours of the day(which is most ideal).

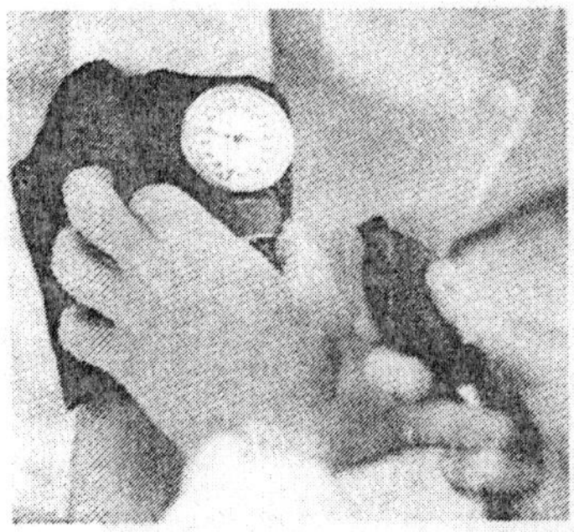

6. Every chemical will give side effects if used in a higher dose. So, for high BP patients - if we are not able to control the BP with a lower dose of one medicine we can add another group of medicine. Since there are about 7-8 groups of Anti hypertension medicines – all with different mechanism of actions- we can combine the medicines to lower their side effects. Such combinations are more preferred than using one particular group of medicine in higher dose.
7. They can be withdrawn and reduced whenever required.
8. They are widely available all over the country, can be carried in a small space, can be taken without a lot of effort (just drink with a glass of water).
9. Most of the allopathic medicines work after about one hour of intake – but in emergency (suppose you are very angry and BP is suddenly 200/100mmHg) there are medicines which can reduce BP within minutes. Intravenous BP lowering drugs are also available.
10. The pattern of medicines, the training of allopathic doctors are uniform all over the world and the country – so you are not dependent on a particular physician or cardiologist. Even if you are in a different city – the allopathic physicians will know your medicines and can modify them.

MONITORING OF YOUR BP DURING TREATMENT

Remember once you have started with the drugs and consume them regularly – you must keep a track of the blood pressure. Keep checking your BP every week for the first few weeks to know that the medicines you have started are working well or not. If it is under controlled or over controlled visit your doctor again for readjustment of medicines.

Once the BP is near 120/80mmHg. It is advised to check your BP less frequently – may be once in a month. I have seen many high BP

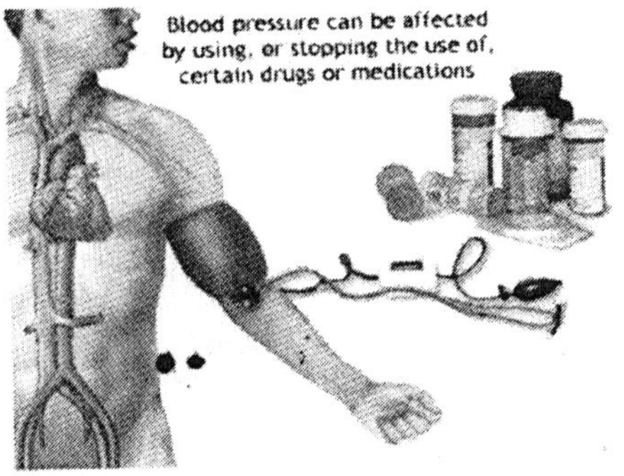

patients who check BP once in a while and even if they find BP high – they do not change the medicines or visit their doctor. This habit is very bad and should be changed.

Remember your BP may vary from day to day, time to time depending on your level of excitement and stress, whether you are checking it after food, exercise or after a sleepless night. So, do not depend on one reading – if you find BP high or very high check it again and again. If they are really high even if you are relaxed – it is time to visit your doctor/physician/cardiologist.

Checking Blood pressure is a very simple procedure and does not take a lot of time. You can get it checked from a local GP or even any health personal (BAMS,BHMS, RMP, Nurse for example). Many people find it difficult to find even such a person I would advice them to buy a BP machine (called Sphygmomanometer) for home use. It must come with a stethoscope and you need to get a training on how to measure the BP. Once you know that you can record them correctly – cross check your reading with a doctor few more times. Now you are ready to check BP at home. It may be difficult to measure your own BP yourself – so get your wife, son, daughter or daughter in law to learn the BP measurement.

Many people find it easy to use the automatic BP instruments – which is also not so bad. But I would definitely want you to cross check the readings with those of a qualified allopathic doctor few times before you start depending on the readings of such electronic devices.

Lastly I would put one word of caution for some people who are stress prone. Such people have a tendency to check BP at home twenty times a day. With every reading they will get worried and the BP will further shoot up. BP can be checked few times in a day only if the BP is higher than 160/100mmHg or if the patient has serious heart disease. For stress prone people it is recommended that they should not be told their reading and it can be recorded by a relative on regular basis – these records will help the doctor to further adjust the dosage.

GROUPS OF BROAD MEDICINES

The drugs which are used to lower BP fall in seven or eight groups – according to the mechanism of actions. I am explaining these groups and discussing these drugs only to make high BP patients understand them and not encouraging self medication. Let all these drugs be prescribed only by an allopathic physician with a minimum qualification of MBBS. But I have seen if the patients also know the details of these drugs – it becomes beneficial and chances of mistakes are very low. It gives a patient satisfaction to know what is he/she consuming and what are they for.

The following are the groups:

a. Beta Blockers
b. Calcium Channel Blockers
c. ACE inhibitors
d. Angiotensin receptor Blockers (ARBs)
e. Diuretics
f. Alpha receptor Blockers
g. Centrally acting drugs
h. Miscellaneous.

Out of these drugs, last three groups are very rarely used. They are used either by old generations of doctors (who have passed MBBS 30-40 years back) or when a particular drug is especially indicated for a particular patient.

Beta blockers (BB) :

Medications that inhibit beta receptors in various parts of the nervous system and the heart, slowdown the heart rate. These help arteries to relax, decrease the force of the heartbeat and reduce blood pressure. Beta blockers are especially useful in patients with heart disease.

Examples (commonly used trade names with company name and dosage):

1. Betaloc – (Astra) -25mg,50mg,100mg
2. Betacard – (Torrent)- 25mg,50mg,100mg
3. Corbis- (unisearch)
4. Aten – (Kopran) – 25mg,50mg,75mg,100mg
5. Atelol- (Thimis)- 25mg,50mg,100mg

6. Tenolol –(IPCA) -12.5mg,25mg,50mg,100mg
7. Seloken XL-(Astra)- 25mg,50mg,100mg
8. Nebicard –(Torrent) – 2.5mg,5mg
9. Metolar- (Cipla)- 25mg,50mg,100mg
10. Concor- (Merck) -5mg,10mg
11. Carca –(Intas)- 3.125mg,6.25mg,12.5mg
12. Cardivas –(Sun pharma) -3.125mg,6.25mg,12.5mg,25mg
13. Atekind – (Mankind) -50mg
14. B.P Norm- (Medley) -25mg,50mg,100mg
15. Carloc – (Cipla) - 3.125mg,6.25mg,12.5mg,25mg
16. Embeta – (Intas) -25mg,50mg,100mg
17. Gudpress-XL –(Mankind) - 25mg,50mg
18. Obeta – (Intas) -25mg,50mg,100mg

Calcium channel blockers (CCB) :

These are a type of vasodilator that inhibit the flow of calcium into heart and blood vessel tissues, reduce tension in the heart, relax blood vessels and lower blood pressure.

Examples:

1. Amlodepin-(Cadila)-2.5mg,5mg,10mg
2. Amlopin-(Sain med.)-2.5mg,5mg,10mg
3. Stamlo-(Dr Reddy's)-2.5mg,5mg,10mg
4. Amlopres-(Cipla)-2.5mg,5mg,10mg
5. Amcard-(Systopic)-2.5mg,5mg,10mg
6. Amlong-(Arsyon)-2.5mg,5mg,7.5mg,10mg
7. Amtas-(Intas)-2.5mg,5mg,10mg
8. Amlosafe-(Gentica)-2.5mg,5mg,10mg
9. Myodura-(Wockhardt)-2.5mg,5mg,10mg
10. Dilzem-(Torrent)-30mg,60mg
11. Angizem-(Sunfarma)-30mg,60mg
12. Calbloc-(Unisearch)-10mg,20mg
13. Depin-(Cadila)-5mg,10mg,20mg
14. Nifedine-(Nicholas)-5mg,10mg
15. Lama-(Stadmen)-5mg,10mg
16. Amlokind-(Mankind)-2.5mg,5mg,10mg

ACE inhibitors (ACE-I) :

These medications are type of vasodilators that help to reduce blood pressure by inhibiting the substances in the blood, that cause blood vessels to constrict. These chemicals called Angiotensinogen groups, are released from the kidneys and if converted to Angiotensin II by a "Converting Enzyme" can increase BP substantially. This group of medicines inhibits ÄCE or Angiotensin Converting Enzyme."

Examples :

1. Listril-(Torrent)-2.5mg.5mg,10mg
2. Lisoril-(Ipca)-2.5mg,5mg,10mg
3. Cipril-(Cipla)-2.5mg,5mg,10mg
4. Envas- H -(Cadila)-10 mg
5. Cardace -(Aventis)-1.25mg,2.5mg.5mg,10mg
6. Repace-(Sunpharma)-25mg,50mg;100mg
7. Ramace-(Astra)-1.25mg,2.5mg.5mg,10mg
8. Covance-(Stancare)-25mg,50mg
9. Coversyl-(Serdia)-2mg,4mg
10. Enace-(Nicholas)-2.5mg,5mg,10mg
11. Captopril-(Wockhardt)-12.5mg,25mg
12. Remipril-(Themis)-1.25mg,2.5mg.5mg,10mg
13. Lipril –(lupin)-2.5mg,5mg,10mg
14. Cardiopril-(Dr Reddy's)-1.25mg,2.5mg.5mg,10mg
15. Losar-(Unisearch)-25mg,50mg

Angiotensin II receptor blockers (ARBs) :

This new class of drugs is showing good results and great promise in reducing hypertension-related complications.

Examples :

1. Losar-(Unisearch)-25mg,50mg
2. Losacar-(Zydus)-25mg,50mg
3. Losakind-(Mankind)-25mg,50mg
4. Losamax-(Indoca)-25mg,50mg

Diuretics:

Medications that promote the formation of urine in the kidneys, causing the body to flush out excess fluids and minerals, especially sodium.

Examples:

1. Lasix-(Aventis)-40mg
2. Ditide-(Glaxo)-50mg
3. Lasilactone-(Aventis)-50mg
4. Amifru (Elder)-40mg
5. Thalizide-(IPCA)-12.5mg

6. Aldactone-(Rpg)-25mg,50mg
7. Dytor-(Cipla)-10mg,20mg,100mg

Alpha blockers (AB):

Medications that inhibit alpha receptors in various parts of the nervous system, slowdown the heart. These help arteries to relax, decrease the force of the heartbeat and reduce blood pressure.

Examples:

1. Minipress-(Pfizer)-2.5mg,5mg
2. Prozopress-(Sunpharma)-1mg,2mg
3. Terapres-(Intas)-1mg,2mg,3mg

Centrally acting drugs

These drugs have the ability to decrease blood pressure without producing sodium retention

1. Methyldopa
   Gynapres- (Mankind) -250mg
2. Clonidine
   Arkamine- (Unisearch)- 100 mcg
   Catapres – (Remedies) -150mcg

Combination of Drugs

To maximize the effectiveness of medicines for reducing BP and minimize the side effects it is very common to combine the anti hypertensive medicines. Different combinations are available. Another advantage of such combination drugs is reduction of the number of tablets to be consumed by the patients – which is always welcome by the patients. Some of the common combination drugs are as follows:

Examples:

1. Amlopress AT (CCB + BB)-Cipla-5+25mg,5+50mg
2. Losar H -ACE-I+ Hydrochlorothiazide) Unisearch- 50mg + 12.5mg
3. Loram-H-(ACE-I+ Hydrochlorothiazide) Unisearch- 50+1.25mg
4. Losar-Beta- (AC-I+ BB)Unisearch-50mg+50mg
5. Ramic-M D.R - John's Lab-(ACE-I+BB)2.5mg + 25mg
6. Repace-A-Sun Pharma-(ACE-I+CCB)25+5mg
7. Amlokind-L-(ACE-I+CCB)-Mankind-5+50mg
8. Adipin Plus-(CCB-BB)-Sain Medicaments-5+50mg

9. Amcard-AT-(CCB-BB)-Systopic-5+50mg
10. Amlo-AT-Pride H.Care-(CCB-BB)-5+50mg
11. Amlokind-(CCB-BB)-AT-Mankind-5+50mg
12. Amlong-A-(CCB-BB)-Caryson-5+50mg
13. Ato Guard-Perk Pharma-(CCB-BB)-5+50+100mg
14. Betabloc-Life Sciences-(CCB-BB)-50+5mg
15. Amace-Systopic-(CCB-ACE-I)-5+5mg
16. Amlopress-L-(CCB-ACE-I)-5+5mg

SIDE EFFECTS OF MEDICINES

Every allopathic medicine has some side effects and I am listing some known side effects of the commonly used groups. But please remember – these side effects only occur in 1-2% cases or very low percentage of patients. You may not be in that class. If, however you notice some side effects you should report to the doctor.

Side effects of Alpha & Beta Blockers : Tiredness, G.I. upset, nightmares, forgetfulness, muscle fatigue, lack of drive, rarely hallucinations.

Side effects of ACE inhibitors : Dry cough, rashes, fall of BP, change in taste sensation, vertigo, headache, bowel upset, anaemia, hyperkalemia (increase in potassium levels above normal)

Side effects of Calcium channel blockers : Constipation, nausea, vertigo, headache, dizziness, flushing, fatigue, nervousness, ankle odema (swelling of ankle), decrease in sensations (due to nervous system involvement.

Side effects of diuretics: Vertigo, visual impairment, calf muscle cramps, anorexia, weakness, giddiness, drowsiness, vomiting, gout, hyperkalemia (potassium more than normal) or hyfokalemia (potassium level less than normal).

SOME COMMON POINTS ON HIGH BP MEDICINES:

1. Please take these allopathic medicines only when you cannot reach a BP level of 130/90 mmHg after following lifestyle changes religiously.
2. Please get these medicines from a qualified Medical doctor with MBBS degree. Do not consult your relatives, local chemist of other pathy (Homoeopathy, Ayurveda or Unani) doctors for High BP medicines.

3. If a particular medicine is not available in the market - you can substitute the medicine with that of another company. But look at the composition of the drug and match them before hand.
4. Many of the medicines which lower the BP are used in heart patients also.
5. **Sudden rise of BP:** Sudden rise of Blood pressure can be caused in High BP patients due to sudden stress. In this case one BP medicine can work to lower the BP immediately. The name of this medicine is Cap. Depin 5mg. and it has to be kept below the tongue. It should be taken only if the BP is above 160/100 mm Hg and after permission from your personal physician.

A DIAGNOSED HYPERTENSIVE MUST

↓

Begin or Continue Lifestyle Modifications

↓

Goal at Blood Pressure (<120/80 mm Hg)
Lower goals for patients with diabetes or renal disease

↓

Initial Drug Choices

Uncomplicated Hypertension	Diuretics, Beta Blockers
Compelling Indications	Diabetes mellitus (type 1) with proteinuria - ACE inhibitors Heart failure - ACE inhibitors, Diuretics Isolated systolic hypertension (older persons) - Diuretics preferred (Older person) - Long - acting dihydropyridine calcium antagonists Myocardial infarction - Beta blockers (non - Isa) ACE inhibitors (with systolic dysfuction)

Start with a low dose of a long - acting, once daily drug, and titrate dose.
Low - dose combinations may be appropriate.

↓

Not at Goal Blood Pressure

↓ No response or troublesome side effects → **Substitute another drug from a different class.**

↓ Indequate but well tolerated → **Add a second agent from a different Class (diuretic if not already used).**

↓

Goal Blood Pressure not achieved

Continue adding agents from other classes.
Consider referral to a hypertension specialist.

Chapter-10

Complications of High Blood Pressure

High blood pressure, if not controlled for a long time leads to many complications. A few of them are:

1. Heart Diseases :

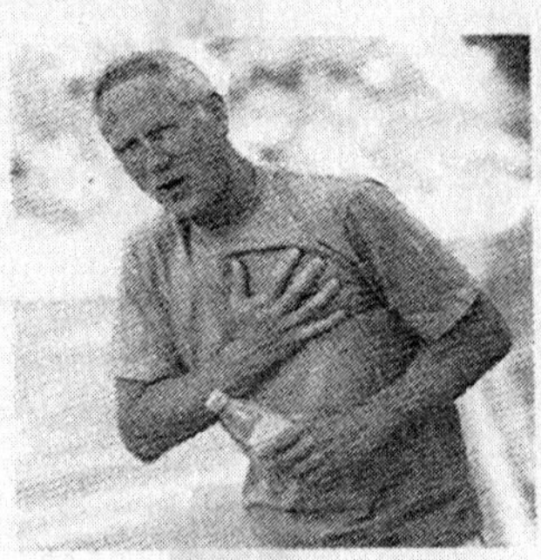

- ☐ Left ventricular hypertrophy i.e enlargement of the left chamber of the heart.
- ☐ Angina
- ☐ Heart Attack (Myocardial infarction)
- ☐ Heart Failure i.e pumping power of heart is decreased & heart is not able to pump blood to organs and muscles. All organs and muscles need oxygen for their proper functioning. This oxygen is supplied through blood. When pumping power of heart decreases these muscles and organs do not get appropriate amount of oxygen.

2. Brain / Nervous Systems

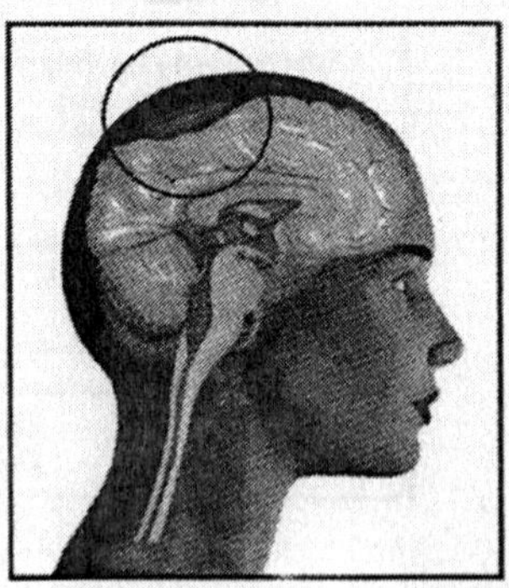

- ☐ **Transient ischemic attack:** Temporary stoppage of blood supply to the brain due to which the patient may develop symptoms like general weakness, weakness in limbs, blindness, numbness These symptoms remain for a few minutes to a few hours.
- ☐ **Stroke:** In this the patient loses her consciousness, develops weakness of

the limbs due to abnormal, severe discharge of blood into the tissue mainly brain, due to occlusion of artery by clot formation in it, or due to rupture of an artery in brain. The patient may go into coma and may die due to other complications.

- **Hypertensive Encephalopathy :** Heart is not able to pump the required blood to brain due to which less oxygen is supplied to it. So due to less supply of oxygen patient becomes irritable, talks irrelevant & complaint of headache.

3. Kidneys:

- Hypertensive Nephropathy : This term includes inflammatory (nephritis) Degenerative and sclerotic (arteriosclerotic) lesions of the kidney, resulting from high pressure in small vessels supplying the kidneys.

4. Eyes :

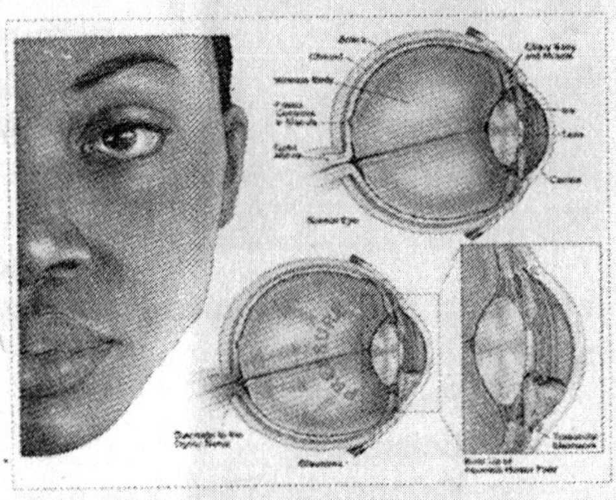

- **Retinopathy :** Retina is the innermost layer of the eye, which aids vision. Hypertension affects retina due to which the patient may lose eyesight.

5. Peripheral arterial diseases:

- Indicates the disease of limbs. Hypertension can cause roughning, stiffness and blockage of these vessels.

If untreated about 50% of hypertension patients die of heart disease, about 33% of stroke and 10-15% of kidney diseases (renal failure). Those with rapidly accelerating hypertension die more frequently of renal failure, as to those who are diabetic, once proteinuria (proteins in urine) or other evidence of kidney diseases develops.

The hypertension induced vascular damage can best be ascertained by examination of eyes, heart and kidney.

Chapter-11

Hypertension Lowering Pregnancy

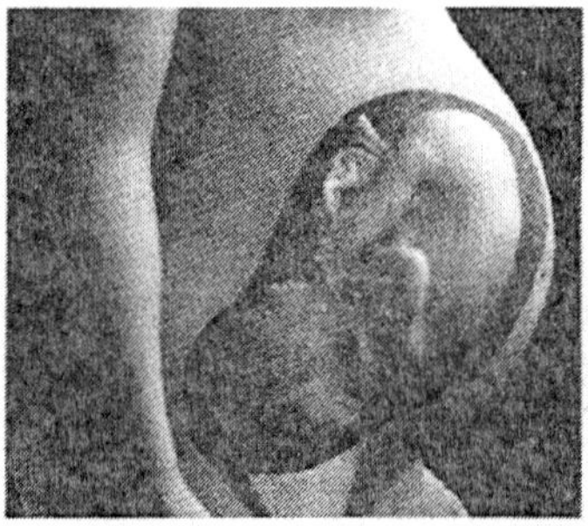

8 to 10% of the population develops hypertension in pregnancy. Pregnancy induced hypertension is defined as a sustained systolic blood pressure of 140 mm Hg or more, and/or a sustained diastolic blood pressure of 90 mm Hg or more.

The word "sustained" here means that the BP is recorded using the same instrument at least 6 hours apart. Pregnancy induced hypertension can be classified as follows:

- Pre-Eclampsia
- Eclampsia

Pre-Eclampsia:-Develops after 20 weeks of pregnancy. There is increase in BP above the normal, together with proteins in urine(more than 0.3grams/litre) and/or generalized swelling of body (general accumulation of fluid in the tissues).

Eclampsia:-If a pregnant woman with high BP, proteins in urine, generalized swelling of the body develops convulsion without any documented brain problem then it is termed as eclampsia.

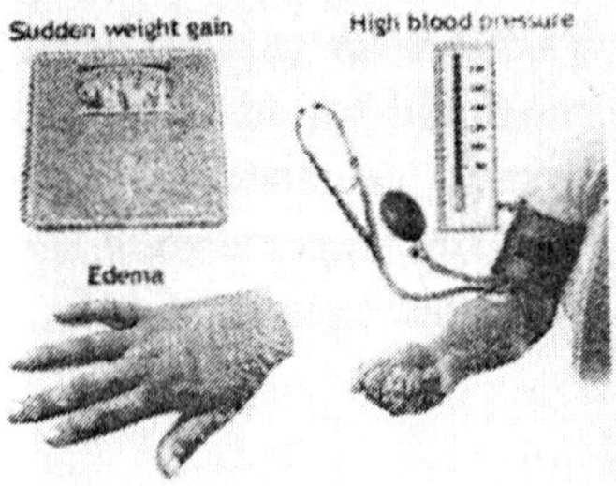

TREATMENT :

The ultimate treatment of this pregnancy induced hypertension is delivery.

❑

Chapter-12

201 Questions or Tips on High Blood Pressure

1. GENERAL QUESTIONS

Q.1. What is blood pressure? Why do we need it?

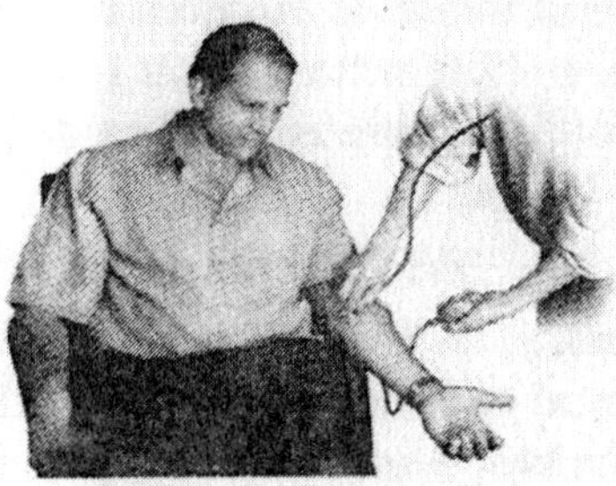

Ans. Our body is supplied with blood, which is equivalent to water of municipal corporation, which supplies water to the whole city. Similarly our heart spreads the blood to the whole body and for this pressure has to be created in all the tubes that go from each part of the body to the heart. All of them are filled up with blood whenever the heart pumps further the blood pressure goes up and this blood pressure spreads the blood to the whole body. This pressure is created in the same way like the municipal corporation water of the city which comes to all the buildings. If the pressure of it is low it will not go to the whole city. Similarly the heart has to pump the blood to spread in the whole body this is why we need the blood pressure.

Q.2. What is normal blood pressure?

Ans. Our normal blood pressure is 120/80mmHg. However, according to the latest research our blood pressure should be 115/75 mmHg.

Q.3. What is hypertension?

Ans. Hypertension is a medical word, which means high blood pressure. When the blood pressure crosses 130/90 mmHg it is termed as hypertension. Hypertension is a very common disease and is found everywhere in the world. In India, the number of hypertensive patients are expected to be 8 to 10% of the adult population.

Q.4. What is the latest figure for normal blood pressure?

Ans. Joint National Committee in 2003 found that the blood pressure is best at 115/75 mmHg. They said that it is even better than the ideal blood pressure which is 120/80 mmHg. Therefore nowadays the normal blood pressure for an adult is considered to be about 115/75 mmHg.

Q.5. What is mmHg?

Ans. mmHg stands for millimeter of the mercury. The blood pressure can be estimated in any form, but it is better to express it as the pressure that can raise the mercury level in a column by millimeter.

Q.6. What is systolic blood pressure?

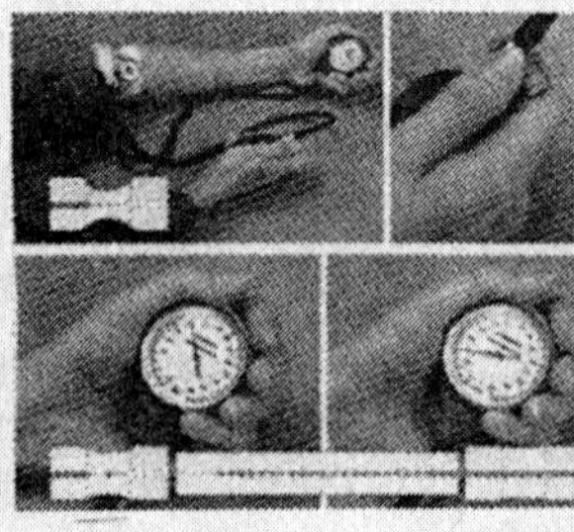

Ans. In our body 5 liters of blood is present. Out of this only 300-400 milliliters of blood is present in the heart and the rest circulates throughout the body. The pure blood which is pumped out from chamber no.4 (left ventricle) is known as systolic blood pressure and it should be 120 mmHg or below.

Q.7. What is diastolic blood pressure?

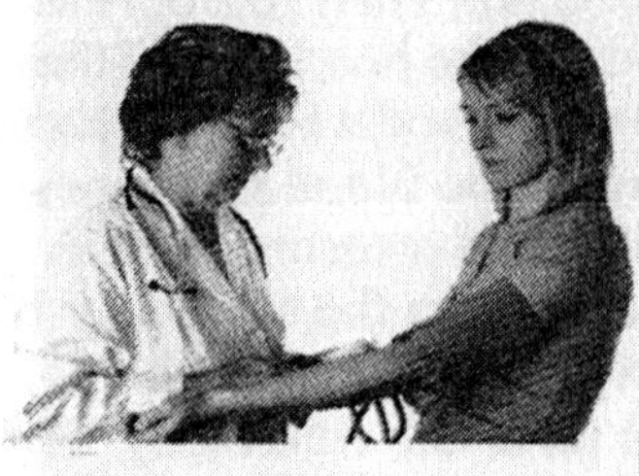

Ans. When the heart relaxes, the blood cannot be pushed in the body. The blood has to be filled up from the body to the heart. At that time the pressure of the blood is not as high as systolic blood pressure. This is the minimum pressure present in the arteries, which is known as diastolic blood pressure. The normal blood pressure is 80mmHg.

Q.8. How is blood pressure measured?

Ans. Blood pressure is measured by using a stethoscope & a blood pressure machine, which is known as sphygmomanometer. Cuff is wrapped around the upper arm over the artery (brachial artery), which supplies blood to the hand. When we inflate the cuff the brachial artery flow gets compressed and after that when we start deflating the cuff slowly by reducing the air pressure, a time comes when the pressure of the blood in the brachial arteries start supplying blood and at that time we can hear a thumping sound that has to be noticed in the meter scale of the blood pressure apparatus. This is known as systolic blood pressure and after some time this sound disappears. The point where the sound disappeares is known as diastolic blood pressure. In this way we can measure the blood pressure.

Q.9. What is meant by mean blood pressure?

Ans. It is the average blood pressure, which is always present in the blood vessels and the tubes of the body. This pressure can be calculated at diastolic +1/3 of the difference between systolic & diastolic blood pressure. Suppose normal blood pressure is 120/80 mmHg. Then the mean blood pressure will be: -

80+1/3(120-80)=80+1/3x40=93.3mmHg.

Q.10. Does Blood pressure differ according to age?

Ans. Yes, in the children the blood pressure is usually low. After the age of 18 we expect the blood pressure to be normal i.e.120/80mmHg. People who do regular exercise, take low salt food, maintain their weight, manage their stress effectively for them, the blood pressure should be 120/80 and below in all ages.

Q.11. What happens in low blood pressure?

Ans. If the blood pressure is low it is unable to supply blood to the whole body. This results in deficiency of blood in every part. In such cases a person may feel weakness, giddiness, and sometimes he may feel like black out.

Q.12. How to diagnose low blood pressure?

Ans. Low blood pressure can be diagnosed by measuring, the blood pressure regularly. If the blood pressure is below 110/70 mmHg then we can call it as low blood pressure. Many men and women have blood pressure in the range of 110/70 mmHg but they do not have any physical symptoms like giddiness etc. In such cases we do not call it as low blood pressure and the treatment is also not required.

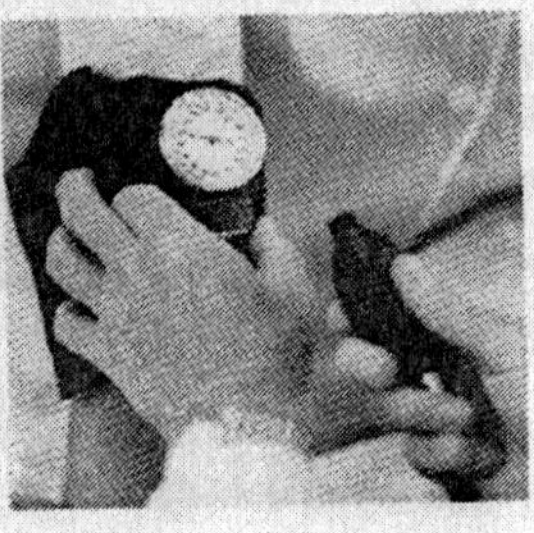

Q.13. What are the grades of hypertension?

Ans. The Grades of high blood pressure are.

	Systolic (mmHg)	Diastolic (mmHg)
Optimal	120 or less	and 80 or less
Normal	129 or less	and 84 or less

High-normal	130-139	and 85-89
Hypertension		
Stage-1	140-159	and 90-99
Stage-2	160-179	and 100-109
Stage-3	180 or higher	and 110 or higher

Q.14. Which blood pressure is more important systolic or diastolic?

Ans. Both systolic and diastolic blood pressures are equally important. However nowadays systolic blood pressure is considered to be more important than the diastolic blood pressure. Earlier it was believed that if the diastolic blood pressure is more than 90mmHg, it damages the body arteries. But now the research has shown that the systolic blood pressure is more important. If it is more than 130 mmHg then prompt treatment should be given. So, never keep the blood pressure above 130mmHg. Ideal blood pressure is 120/80mmHg.

Q.15. What is labile hypertension?

Ans. In patients with stress or anxiety, blood pressure suddenly rises above 200mmHg. It is also known as labile hypertension. This type of hypertension usually occurs due to stress.

Q.16. What is pre-hypertension?

Ans. Pre-hypertension is the stage in which the blood pressure rises to a very small extent. Pre-hypertension is also known as stage1 hypertension, occurs due to metabolic syndrome. In pre-hypertension the blood pressure should be below 140/90mmHg. Pre-hypertension does not need any medication. It can be controlled by diet and exercises.

Q.17. What is JNC? On what basis do they change the grading of hypertension?

Ans. JNC means Joint National Committee. It is a center, formed by the cardiologists all over the world. This committee has to produce new researches every year. Till now JNC has given seven studies of hypertension and the last study showed that blood pressure should be 115-75mmHg in all ages. This committee also advises life style modification, diet control, regular exercises to keep the blood pressure in the latest normal range.

Q.18. Many doctors still believe blood pressure of 140/90mmHg is normal. Is it ok?

Ans. No, it is not ok. Some times doctors do not get the latest information of the new studies. According to older studies the blood pressure 140/90 mmHg was considered to be normal. Many doctors treat the patients according to the old research and say 140/90mmHg blood pressure according to age is normal.

Q.19. There was dictum that the systolic blood pressure is age+ 100. Is it correct?

Ans. No, it is not correct. Earlier it was said that the blood pressure rises with age. At that time a blood pressure of 150 mmHg at the age of 50 was considered as normal. But the dictum has now, changed. Now the blood pressure should remain the same that is 120/80 mmHg at all ages. Even at the age of 70 the ideal blood pressure should be 120/80 mmHg.

2. DIAGNOSIS, SIGNS & SYMPTOMS

Q.20. What are the sounds that we hear while measuring blood pressure with the stethoscope?

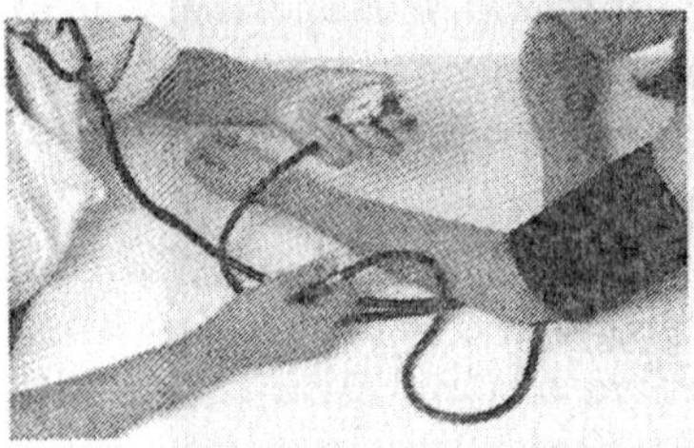

Ans. While measuring blood pressure by stethoscope we hear a thumping sound, which continues for sometime and then disappears. The point at which the thumping sound starts is the systolic blood pressure and the sound at which it disappears is diastolic blood pressure.

Q.21. Can we measure blood pressure without stethoscope?

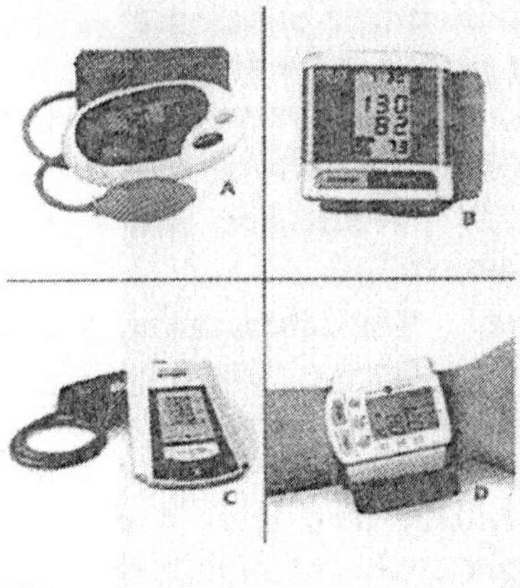

Ans. Yes, we can measure blood pressure without stethoscope. But only the systolic blood pressure can be measured & the readings will be approximate. For this before inflating the cuff on the brachial artery we have to find out the brachial artery near the wrist. After that you have to inflate the cuff above systolic pressure and air is then slowly released. The first movement when we feel the artery, that is systolic blood pressure. The reading can then be noted from the mercury column.

Q.22. Can we measure our own blood pressure by using stethoscope & blood pressure machine? Can my family member measure it?

Ans. Yes, we can measure our blood pressure by using stethoscope. The only problem that surfaces in this case is to tie the cuff on the elbow. However, some special types of cuffs are also available which one can easily put on his own. If the cuff is placed in the right position then it is not difficult to check the blood pressure and even your family members can check it. They only need to learn the procedure for measuring blood pressure correctly.

Q.23. What are the kinds of blood pressure apparatus available in the market? Which one is better?

Ans. There are three kinds of blood pressure machines.

1. Mercury manometer.
2. Dial type manometer.
3. Electronic blood pressure apparatus.

Among these, mercury manometer and dial type manometer are more authentic. In electronic machine there is always an error of 5.6 millimeter of mercury. So, we get approximate reading by using this apparatus. Electronic blood pressure apparatus are also of two types: in one type you have to fix the cuff on the arms and push the buttons, whereas the other type is like your wristwatch to be worn on the wrist. Before buying the electronic apparatus one must compare it's reading with that of the manual blood pressure apparatus to avoid the error.

Q.24 What happens during high blood pressure?

Ans. During high blood pressure, one usually complains of headache and their face colour may also change to red. But it is usually seen that the people with headache do not try to measure their blood pressure and when they measure it they find it high. As such high blood pressure shows no specific symptoms.

Q.25. What are the causes of high blood pressure?

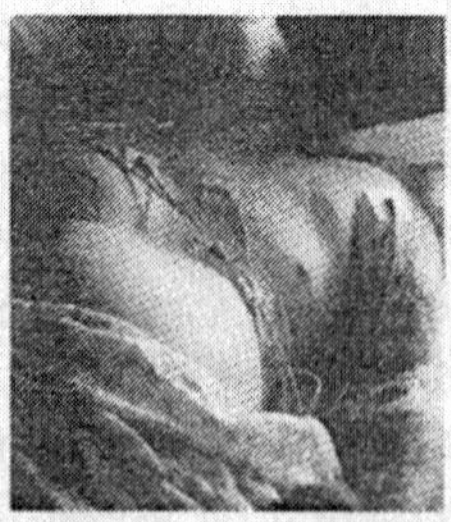

Ans. The actual cause of high blood pressure is still not known. But it is believed that stress plays a very important role in the development of hypertension. However, obesity, lack of exercises, heredity and diet are also responsible for hypertension or high blood pressure.

For example, if husband and wife have different viewpoints and they do not agree with each other's view, then there will be clashes. In other words, if we do not get what we want fight may occur. To avoid this, one has to understand the other person's mind. This is called Anekant. Anekant means every person has different opinion. One must accept this and show respect towards the other person's view and should not fight.

Q.137. How can financial stress be managed?

Ans. Money plays an important role in everyone's life. For example- for every want or activity one needs money. So balancing the money sector is very important. Nowadays, most of the people are stressed due to financial problem. This is because they spend more than their income. But if they could manage to control expenditure or if their expenditure is less than their income, the financial stress will immediately disappear. But if their expenditure increases than their income, the stress will also increase. To reduce stress, it is necessary to strike a balance between income and expenditure.

Saving is another way of managing stress. If one saves a small percent of this income; it will help him in case of need. Thus, saving also helps to reduce financial stress in emergency situations.

Q.138. Do satsangs help to reduce stress?

Ans. Yes. Our subconscious mind is full of good things. By visiting satsang you may continuously remember what things are good or how to behave. Such satsangs are beneficial, if one hears everyday, and tries to apply them in your daily life, to live a peaceful and happy life, we need lot of advice which we already know. But in satsang, when we hear them again and again, it changes our mind and helps to apply them in our life.

Q.139. How can we control Ego?

Ans. Ego makes people feel, that they are good or superior to others. This leads to a lot of stress, if they fail to prove their superiority. So, to reduce ego a person should try to find out his bad qualities and other people's good qualities. But if you see the bad qualities of others, then you feel yourself superior. And if you feel the good qualities of other, then you can understand that your ego is not justified. So, to cut down ego you have to understand a term known as Harmony- in Hindi it means Har—mani. If you understand your own fault and know that

any defect in endocrine system. But along with this patient should also measure their blood sugar level, serum cholesterol, and triglyceride, which also raise the blood pressure and leads to coronary blockages. Urine test and total blood count can be done. Electro-cardiogram must be done in all high blood pressure patients & X-ray to rule out an enlargement of heart etc.

Q.32. What is ambulatory blood pressure measurement?

Ans. The blood pressure of certain individuals goes up when they visit a doctor. But while sleeping or relaxing their blood pressure is normal. So, such people are usually advised to wear a portable device known as ambulatory blood pressure machine. It is a small portable machine, which is worn on the body, and takes the reading of your blood pressure throughout the day, and if the readings are high then it is diagnosed as high blood pressure. This is ambulatory blood pressure measurement.

Q. 33. Which blood pressure machine is better: mercury type or dial type?

Ans. Mercury type blood pressure apparatus is better than dial type. Earlier, doctors were using the mercury apparatus only but due to inconvenience in carrying this apparatus, the dial type blood pressure apparatus is commonly used nowadays.

Q. 34. Can we depend on the readings of our electronic blood pressure machines?

Ans. It is not so that electronic blood pressure machines do not give accurate blood pressure reading. But one must be careful while buying the electronic machines. They must make sure that there is no error in the apparatus.

Q. 35. How often can blood pressure be measured?

Ans. The people who have normal blood pressure can measure their blood pressure once in a month, but the people with high blood pressure or cardiac problem (heart disease) should measure their blood pressure more frequently. Those who have very high blood pressure should be measured daily to monitor their blood pressure. Whenever you are starting the drugs you should keep monitoring the blood pressure on regular basis. But blood pressure should not be measured on hourly basis.

3. TREATMENT OF HYPERTENSION

Q.36. What should be the aim of treating blood pressure?

Ans. The main aim of treating blood pressure is to reduce the blood pressure level and to keep it below 120/80 mmHg. If the blood pressure is not very high (more than 140/90 mmHg), then it can also be controlled by diet modification (low salt diet), regular exercises and by stress management. But if the blood pressure is still high then the drugs must be started to reduce the blood pressure.

Q.37. How to treat hypertension?

Ans. Hypertension can be treated in many ways. If the blood pressure is slightly higher than normal, then it can be treated by a low salt diet, avoiding alcohol, smoking and reducing the level of stress. Regular exercise and meditation also help in reducing the blood pressure. But, if the blood pressure is more than 130/90 mmHg, then one must also start taking medicines along with diet modification and exercises.

Q. 38. What role does medicine play in hypertension?

Ans. There are several ways in which hypertensive medicines help to reduce the blood pressure. For instance, some of these medicines act by stopping the leakage of calcium ions in the arteries. They also act by stopping the secretion of angiotensin hormone, extracting sodium from blood etc, thereby helping to keep the blood pressure within the normal range. For this it is also necessary to continue the medicines for a long time.

Q.39. Which medicines can be used in hypertension?

Ans. Hypertension is a very common disease nowadays. Many people with mild hypertension don't even know that they are hypertensive. But the people who know that their blood pressure is high can take medicines for reducing the blood pressure. The group of medicines that are in use to treat hypertension are Alpha and Beta- blockers, calcium channels blockers, ACE Inhibitors, Diuretics – AngiotensinII receptor blockers, Central acting agent and direct vasodilators.

Q.40. What are diuretics? Give some examples?

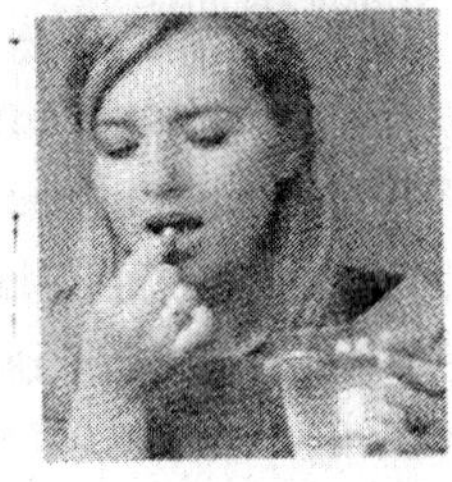

Ans. Diuretics refer to the drugs that help in reducing the volume of fluid in the body. These medicines for reducing the blood pressure are very commonly used nowadays. They help to excrete more sodium in the urine. Sodium removes water from the blood thereby reducing the volume of blood pushing through the arteries. This decrease in blood volume also leads to a fall in blood pressure. Some commonly used diuretics are:

1. Thiazides: Diuril, Hygroton, Oretic, Diulo Zaroxolyn.
2. Loop (extract sodium in large amount): lasix, edecrin, bumex, demadex.
3. Potassium sparing: Midamor, Aldactone, Dyrenium

Diuretics help to extract both sodium and potassium whereas potassium sparing group of diuretics only extract sodium from the blood.

Q.41. What are Beta-blockers? Give some examples?

Ans. Beta blockers help to lower the blood pressure by blocking the effects of the hormone called nor-epinephrine (nor-adrenaline). They also reduce the impulse of beta-receptors present in the heart, which makes the heart beat faster and the blood vessels to contract and expand. This drug was earlier used to treat coronary heart disease but later on it was found to be more effective in treating hypertension. Examples: Tenormin, Inderal, Tenolol, Atecad, Aten, Betacard.

Q.42. What are alpha-blockers? Give some examples?

Ans. Alpha blockers help to reduce the effects of the non-adrenaline and adrenaline hormones in the body. These hormones narrow the blood vessels and make the heart to work more. If the heart rate increases, the blood pressure also increases. Alpha-blockers also improve the flow of urine, which is useful for the patient with prostate problem. Examples are: Hytrin, Cardura, Minipress etc.

Q.43. What are calcium channel blockers? Give some examples?

Ans. Our body contains many cells having small channels (passages) called calcium channels. When calcium flows into these channels the cells of the muscles contract and the arteries narrow, which increases the blood pressure. And if the leaking process of calcium stops the arteries will relax and allow the blood to flow smoothly thereby reducing the blood pressure.

Examples: Amcard, Amdepin, Amlo, Amlodac, Amlopres, Amlovas,

Q.44. What are ACE inhibitors? Give some examples?

Ans. Ace Inhibitors refer to angiotensin converting enzymes. Angiotensin is made up of two words Angio –blood vessels and tensin-

pressure. Angiotensin is a substance, which contracts (narrows) the blood vessels and increases the blood pressure. ACE inhibitors help to reduce the production of angiotensin from its precursor called angiotensinogen and allow the blood to flow smoothly. Examples are: Ramace, Listil, Enace, Envas, Aceten, Capotril.

Q.45.. What are Angiotensin II receptor blockers? Give some examples?

Ans. Angiotensin II receptor blocker is a new class of drugs that can be used to control hypertension. This drug also blocks the formation of angiotensin in the body.

Some examples: Losar, Losar-H, Losacor, Repace, Tozaar, Repace-H.

Q.46. What are central acting agent drugs? Give some examples?

Ans. Central acting agent drugs prevent the brain from sending signals to the nervous system to increase the heart rate and narrow the blood vessels. Some of the central acting agent drugs are Arkamin, Catapress, Tenex, Aldemet, Serpasil.

Q.47. What are vaso dilators? Give some examples?

Ans. Vasodilators refers to a group of drugs, which are used to treat severe hypertensives that are not responding to any other hypertensive medicines. These drugs directly act on the muscles wall of the arteries and prevent them from tightening and narrowing.

Examples of vasodilators are: Cardif, Nitrepin, Felogaris, Calcigard, Depin, Myogard, Nifedine.

Q.48. How to tackle hypertension in an emergency?

Ans. Anti hypertension drugs like calcium channel blockers, beta-blockers, ACE inhibitors are taken orally and they take about 30minutes to come in contact with the blood. So they cannot be used in case of an emergency. Therefore in an emergency it is always advisable to make the patient relax and then give him a medicine of this group to keep under the tongue. This will help to reduce the blood pressure immediately. The patient can also be given anti-anxiety injection to make him feel relaxed. This also helps to reduce the blood pressure.

Q.49. How long should the medication for lowering the blood pressure continue?

Ans. Hypertension medicines must be taken for a considerable period of time. Many times people think that the medicines if taken regularly for 10-15 days will cure the disease permanently. But unfortunately these medicines only help in controlling the blood pressure and maintaining it within the normal range. However, once the blood pressure is controlled the dosage can be reduced.

Q.50. Do hypertension drugs have side effects?

Ans. All allopathic drugs have some side effects. Inspite of this a high blood pressure patient must take these medicines to keep the blood pressure under control.

Q.51. What are the side effects of diuretics?

Ans. If the diuretics are taken in a high dosage they can cause weakness or dizziness. They may also result in a high blood sugar, cholesterol and uric acid level. It also increases the chances of developing gout in future.

Q.52. What are the side effects of Beta-blockers?

Ans. Beta-blockers have more side effects than the other blood pressure medicines. The side effects include fatigue, cold hands, sleeping trouble, loss of sex drive and a slight increase in the triglyceride level.

However for severe asthmatic patients and beta-blockers are not recommended.

Q.53. What are the side effects of ACE inhibitors?

Ans. The side effects of ACE inhibitors are dry cough, rashes, altered sense of taste and reduced appetite. This group of drugs is not recommended for severe kidney disease patients.

Q.54. What are the side effects of Angiotensin II receptor blockers?

Ans. Angiotensin II receptor blockers have very minimum side effects. But they may cause dizziness, nasal congestion, leg pain, back pain, diarrhoea, indigestion and insomnia. Angiotensin II receptor blockers are not recommended for severe kidney disease patients and during pregnancy.

Q.55. What are the side effects of alpha-blockers?

Ans. The side effects of alpha-blockers are headache, nausea, weakness, and reduced heart rate.

Q.56. What are the side effects of central-acting agents?

Ans: Central-acting agents can cause fatigue, drowsiness or sedation, dry mouth, headache, weight gain and psychological problems like depression.

Q.57. What are the side effects of vasodilators?

Ans. Vasodilators may cause gastrointestinal problem, dizziness, headache, nasal congestion, and excessive hair growth all over the body and swelling of the gums.

Q.58. Is it safe to take hypertension drugs in long term?

Ans. Yes, it is safe to take hypertension drugs in long term because the hypertension medicine helps to keep the blood pressure low. It also has minimum side effects. So, blood pressure medicines can be taken in a long run to control the blood pressure.

Q.59. Can these drugs be combined together?

Ans. Yes, these drugs can be combined together. Many a times a single drug is not able to control the blood pressure. In such cases if the dosage is increased, the risk of side effects will also increase. Therefore, it is always better to use a combination of drugs, which will help to control the blood pressure with minimum side effects.

Q.60. Can the medicines for blood pressure be stopped at any time in one's life?

Ans. Yes, blood pressure medicines can be stopped if the blood pressure comes down to 120/80 or below. But before stopping the medicines, one must make sure that the blood pressure does not increase without medicines. One must also regularly do yoga, exercise and meditation, which will help to reduce the blood pressure.

So, if one is doing regular meditation, yoga and exercise and maintaining the blood pressure below 120/80 mmHg, then the medicines can be stopped.

Q.61. Do we need to reduce these medicines once the blood pressure comes down to 120/80mmHg or below?

Ans. Yes, we can reduce the medicines if the blood pressure comes down to 120/80mmHg or below. But if the blood pressure increases after the dosage is reduced, it means the normal blood pressure was due to the action of drugs. So, in such cases, the medicines cannot be reduced.

Q.62. What to do if the blood pressure is 120/80mmHg?

Ans. Blood pressure, 120/80 mmHg is a normal reading. If the blood pressure is 120/80 mmHg, then one must try to maintain this blood pressure in future also. It can be maintained by doing regular exercise; yoga, meditation and taking proper diet. Stress is one of the main causes of high blood pressure and it must also be controlled to keep the blood pressure within normal limits.

Q.63. What to do if the blood pressure goes down below 120/80 mm Hg?

Ans. If the blood pressure goes slightly below120/80 mmHg, there is nothing to worry about. It may be due to the action of antihypertensive drugs in the body. But if the blood pressure goes very low (90/60mmHg) with physical symptoms like giddiness and weakness, then the dosage of medicine must be reduced. However, if the person is not taking any blood pressure medicines then he should take a cup of coffee or tea, which will help to increase the blood pressure.

4. DIET AND HYPERTENSION

Q.64. Can a hypertensive patient use salt in food preparation?

Ans. There are two kinds of hypertensive patients-salt sensitive and salt insensitive. In both the cases some amount of salt restriction is necessary. However if you are salt insensitive then, you can use salt in food preparation but no salt at the table is allowed.

Q.65. What is salt sensitive hypertension?

Ans. There are two kinds of hypertensive patients-salt sensitive and salt insensitive. Salt sensitive patients are those, whose blood pressure is affected with salt intake. An intake of a small amount of salt leads to a sudden rise in their blood pressure, whereas salt restriction helps to lower the blood pressure in these patients. Therefore, these patients must restrict salt in their diet.

Q.66. What is salt insensitive hypertension?

Ans. Salt insensitive hypertensives are those who are not sensitive towards salt. Salt intake or restriction has no effect on their blood pressure. To find out whether you are salt sensitive or not, consume a diet containing normal amounts of salt regularly for 4-5 days. At the same time, you must also keep a check on your blood pressure. If you notice any rise in your blood pressure with the salt intake it means you are salt sensitive, and you must restrict salt in your diet. However, if no change in blood pressure occurs it indicates that you are salt insensitive and you can consume normal amount of salt but no salt at the table should be taken.

Q.67. How does high fiber diet help to reduce hypertension?

Ans. Taking high fiber diet helps to reduce triglycerides and cholesterol levels. Fiber also helps to control diabetes and aids in weight reduction. Obesity and diabetes are the risk factors for hypertension and controlling the risk factors can ultimately lead to lowering of blood pressure.

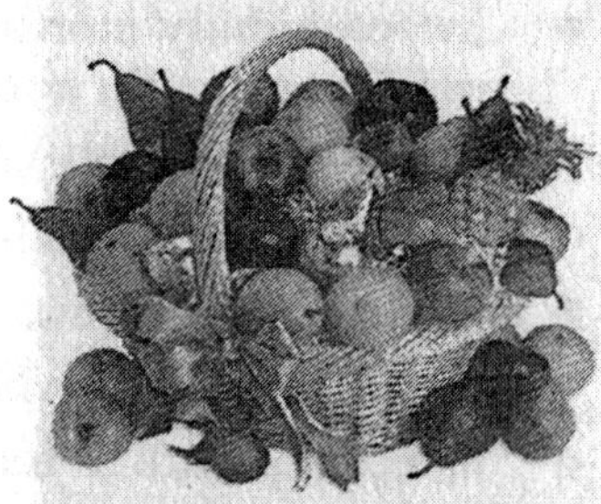

Q.68. Can I take tea/coffee more than 1-2 times in a day?

Ans. Coffee is a stimulating beverage, which increases your heart rate thereby increasing your blood pressure. Therefore strong tea or coffee is usually recommended to a hypotensive patient. Taking 1-2 cups of tea or coffee in a day is not harmful but it must never be consumed in excess.

Q.69. Can a high cholesterol diet increase the blood pressure?

Ans. Yes, a high cholesterol diet will definitely increase your blood pressure. The dietary cholesterol over the years gets deposited in the arteries supplying blood to the heart and the rest of the body. As a result of this the space available for the blood in the arteries become less and this increases the blood pressure due to atherosclerosis (blockage) in coronary artery. Blockage in other arteries also increases the blood pressure.

Q.70. What do you mean by Dash Diet?

Ans. The DASH (Dietary Approaches to Stop Hypertension) diet emphasizes on fruits, green vegetables, and low-fat dairy products. It also includes small amounts of fish, poultry, and nuts; and reduces consumption of red meat and sweets. It also reduces the level of salt intake. The DASH diet is also high in fiber and protein.

Q.71. What are the basic advice by Dash Diet?

Ans. Following advice are given by Dash:

- Consume a variety of foods within and among the basic food groups while staying within energy needs.
- Control calorie intake to manage body weight.

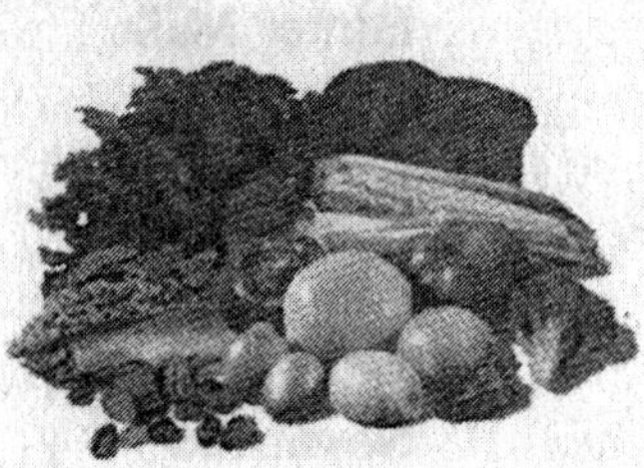

- Do physically active work every day.
- Increase daily intake of fruits and vegetables, whole grains, and nonfat or low-fat milk and its products.
- Choose fats wisely for good health.
- Choose carbohydrates wisely for good health.
- Choose and prepare foods with little salt.
- If you drink alcoholic beverages, do so in moderation.
- Keep food safe to eat.

Q.72. What is a combination diet?

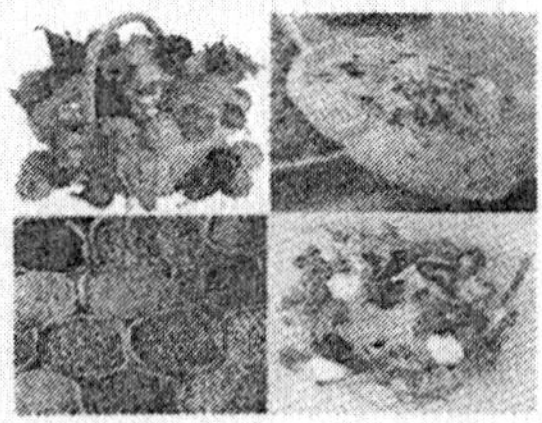

Ans. Combination diet includes fresh fruits, vegetables, ample amount of grains and very low fat dairy products. According to this diet fat intake should be less than 30% of total calories.

Q.73. Why combination diet is considered useful for hypertension patient?

Ans. It is seen that hypertensive people who are on combination diet experience an average decrease of 11.4mmHg in systolic and 5.5mmHg in diastolic pressure. This effect is similar to the one that is produced by the use of medications.

Q.74. Why combination diet is better in hypertension patient?

Ans. Combination diet is better in hypertension patient because it is rich in potassium, calcium and magnesium.

Q.75. What are the sources of Calcium?

Ans. The optimal calcium intake of adults should be 400 mg/day. Here are the foods that can help you reach that amount. The best sources of Calcium are:

Calcium (milligrams)	per 100 gms:
Skimmed Milk	120
Butter Milk	30
Ragi	344
Chana	202
Moth	202
Rajma	260
Soyabean	240

Maa ki dal	154
Bathua leaves	150
Cauliflower	626
Coriander leaves	184
Curry leaves	830
Methi leaves	395
Sarson	155
Salad leaves	320
Raddish leaves	280
Palak	75
Carrot	80
Onion	50
Radish	70
Beans	50
Lady finger	66
Kamal Kakri	405
Amla	50
Bael	85
Khajoor	120
Munakka	130
Angeer	80
Guava	50
Lemon	70
Phalsa	129
Kishmish	90
Cane Jaggery	80
Date Jaggery	363

Q.76. What are the sources of Magnesium?

Ans. Magnesium is found in a wide variety of foods and in drinking water. Regularly eating green leafy vegetables, whole grains and legumes will ensure you get an adequate amount. It is also found in small amounts in animal products e.g. meat, fish and poultry. However, a hypertensive patient must not consume them.

Q.77. What are the sources of Potassium?

Ans. The following foods have moderate to very high amount of potassium in each serving.

Asparagus(Chaulai),Broccoli, Carrots, Corn (Bhutta) Beans, Banana, Peas, Turnips (Shalgam), Mushrooms (Khumbi), Potatoes, Pumpkin (Kaddu), Spinach (Palak), Sweet potatoes, Tomato, Apple, Black berries (Jamun), Cherries, Peaches (Aadoo), Pear (Nashpati), Fresh Pineapple, Raisins (Kishmish), Raspberries, Apricots (Khumani), Dates (Khajoor), Guava, Mango, Orange, Prunes (Munnakka), Strawberries, Watermelon, Papayas.

Q.78. What are anti-oxidants?

Ans: Anti-oxidants act as cell protectors. Anti-oxidants are nutrients (vitamins and minerals) as well as enzymes (protein in your body that assists in chemical reactions). They protect the body against the destructive effects of free radicals. Anti-oxidants counteract these free radicals and bind with them before they can cause damage. If left unchecked, free radicals may cause heart damage, cancer, and high blood pressure.

There are three types of anti-oxidants. -

1) Vitamin A
2) Vitamin C
3) Vitamin E

Q.79. What are the sources of anti-oxidants?

Ans: Anti-oxidants are found in

1) Vitamin A:-green leafy vegetables, fruits (coloured), vegetables.

2) Vitamin C:-amla, orange, guava, mausambi, green chilli.

3) Vitamin E:- sprouts, all cereals and pulses.

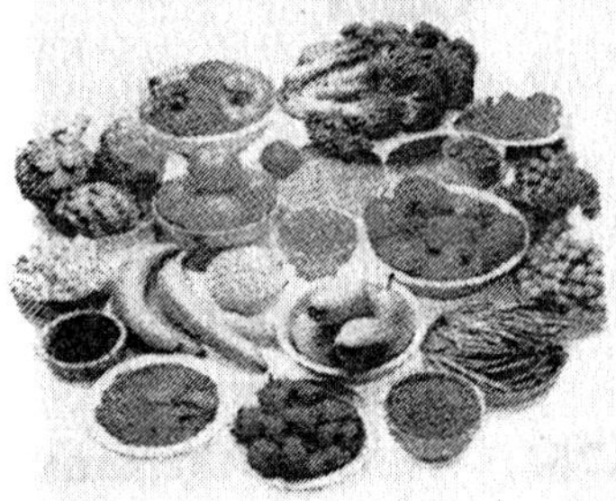

Q.80. Do anti-oxidants also help in hypertension?

Ans: Yes, anti-oxidants do help in hypertension because together, these nutrients form a powerful alliance that can help to protect the body from many diseases specially heart diseases and hypertension.

Vitamin C- is a powerful anti-oxidant. It cleans the body impurities and improves iron absorption.

Vitamin E- is a potent cleanser and a powerful antioxidant. It also cleans the body impurities and helps in lowering high cholesterol. It also reduces narrowing of the arteries and also hypertension.

5. OBESITY AND HYPERTENSION

Q.81. How is obesity responsible for hypertension?

Ans. It has been seen that obese people generally have a high blood pressure. This is because in obese people the peripheral resistance i.e. the resistance of the arteries to blood flow is more which is responsible for high blood pressure.

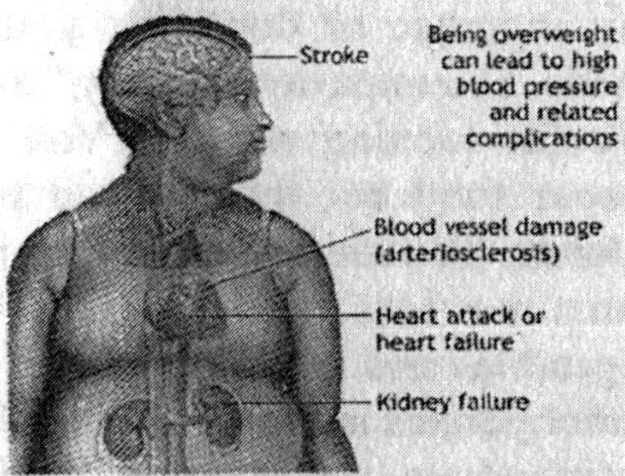

Weight reduction in obese individuals also help in controlling blood pressure. It has been seen that with a reduction of 1-2 kg of weight the blood pressure also drops by 1 –2 mm Hg.

Q.82. How to rule out the obesity of a person?

Ans. Obesity of a person can be detected by seeing the ratio of weight according to height. For that, there are standard charts available from where one can find out whether he is obese or not. In India, LIC charts are available, where the information about weight and height relationship is given.

Q.83. What is BMI?

Ans. BMI (Body Mass Index) is the scientific way of measuring obesity. It is a number based on both your height and weight. It can help you determine the degree to which you may be overweight and gives a reasonable assessment of total body fat for the general population.

18.5 to 24.9	=	Healthy Weight
25 to 29.9	=	Over Weight
30 to 34.9	=	Obesity (Class I)
35 to 39.9	=	Obesity (Class 2)
40 or more	+	Severe Obesity (Class 3)

For example, if the person's weight is 52 kg and Height is 1.65 meter

Weight (kg)/Height (meter^2) =52/ $(1.65)^2$= 19

Q.84. How can I reduce weight?

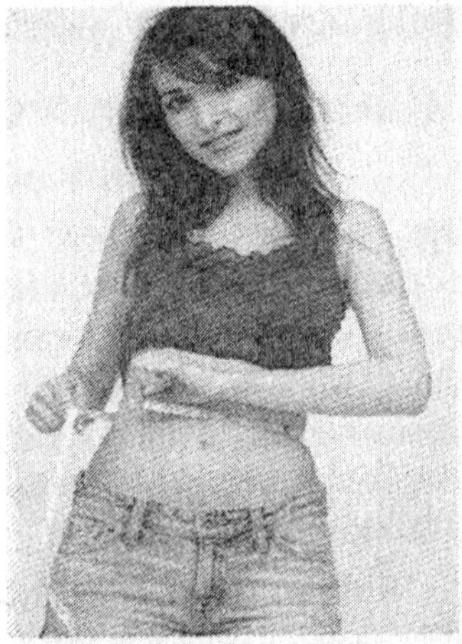

Ans. The reduction of weight is not very difficult. It is the balance between the calories intake and calories expenditure.Diet modification can help you increase or decrease your calorie intake. You must never apply **"not to eat"** rule for loosing weight. You must eat proper food but that should be of low calories. To reduce weight you must also consume lots of fibrous fruits and vegetables and include more of complex carbohydrates in the diet instead of simple carbohydrate. An obese individual must also avoid fruits like banana, cheeku, grapes and mango. You must also do regular exercise or walk but should not eat high calorie food after that. Instead, you can take fresh fruits and juices.

Q.85. How can you differentiate overweight and obesity?

Ans. The difference between overweight and obesity is a matter of degree. Federal guidelines define overweight as having a body mass index (BMI) between 25 to 29. Obesity is between 30-35.

Q.86. In addition to high blood pressure what other disease does obesity lead to?

Ans. Obesity significantly increases risk for:- Diabetes, Heart Disease, Stroke and Cervical Cancer(in females).

Q.87. Does BMI differ in male & female?

Ans. Unlike weight & height tables, BMI doesn't differ between men & women.

6. HYPERTENSION & CORONARY ARTERY DISEASE/ MYOCARDIAL INFARCTION

Q.88. What is Coronary Artery Disease?

Ans. Coronary Artery Disease (CAD) means blockages in the coronary arteries, or in other words we can say that the arteries supplying blood to the heart muscles get blocked. In such cases the patients feel typical chest pain on the left side. This pain is called angina. This angina increases on walking fast and decreases on taking rest. In angina, patient may also feel heaviness in chest, palpitation or burning sensation in the chest. Such people are very liable to develop heart attack(Myocardial Infarction) in the later phase of their life.

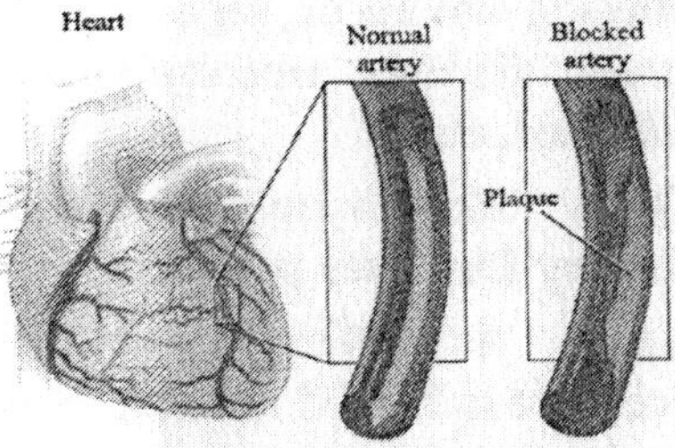

Q.89. What is Myocardial Infarction?

Ans. In a coronary heart patient there is 70% blockage in the coronary arteries. But if this blockage is more than 80% or 90%, the heart does not get adequate blood especially at the time of exercise. At this time the patient feels pain. Myocardial Infarction is one of the complications of coronary heart disease. In this the membrane covering the coronary arteries gets ruptured releasing some chemicals leading to clotting of blood in these arteries. So, if the blockage is already 80% and the remaining 20-30% gets filled up with the clot then the tubes will become 100% blocked and this will lead to death or damage of the heart muscles supplied by the coronary arteries.

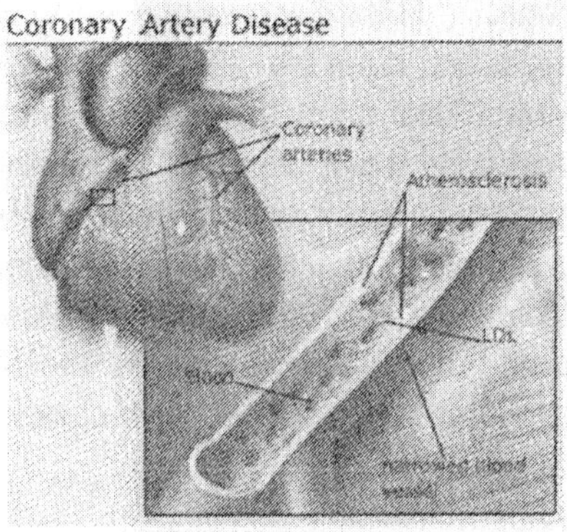

Q.90 How is hypertension responsible for CAD/MI?

Ans. Due to high blood pressure the arteries supplying blood to the heart get narrowed, and the blood cannot pass easily through them. Deficiency in blood and oxygen to the coronary arteries leads to heart attack. So, to avoid the risk of CAD one should try to keep the blood pressure in normal range, that is 120/80mmHg or below.

Q.91. Is only hypertension responsible for development of coronary Heart disease?

Ans. No.There are other 14-15 risk factors, which also can lead to coronary heart disease. They are high cholesterol, high triglycerides, obesity, low HDL, high LDL cholesterol : HDL ratio, LDL:HDL ratio, stress, diabetes, obesity, smoking, lack of fiber, lack of antioxidants ,alcohol, etc.

Q.92. How much Blood Pressure is safe for CAD (Coronary Artery Disease) patients?

Ans. According to joint national committee, 2003 the ideal blood pressure is 115/75 mmHg. However, a blood pressure of 120/80mmHg is also considered safe for coronary artery disease patients. But if your blood pressure is more than 120/80 mmHg you're at risk of developing other cardiac diseases.

Q.93. How to control the blood pressure in a coronary artery disease patient?

Ans. Blood pressure is a silent killer.In a normal person blood pressure rises by 2%per year and in hypertensives it rises by 4%per year.If the blood pressure is not in control,it increases the chances of coronary heart disease. Therefore, in order to control the blood pressure and maintain it within normal limits you must try to reduce your weight, cut down on your stress and do yoga, meditation, walking everyday. You must also eat high fiber, low cholesterol and low fat food. If, inspite of all the above measures the blood pressure is not controlled then the drugs must be started and continued until a good blood pressure control is achieved. .

7. HYPERTENSION & STROKE /CVA

Q.94. How does hypertension lead to stroke/CVA?

Ans. Increase in blood pressure increases the pressure in the cerebral arteries by which they become weaker and weaker and ultimately these arteries burst causing cerebral embolism or cerebral hemorrhage. This in turn will lead to death of the brain. In more than 50% of the cases, cerebral vascular accident or stroke occurs due to high blood pressure.

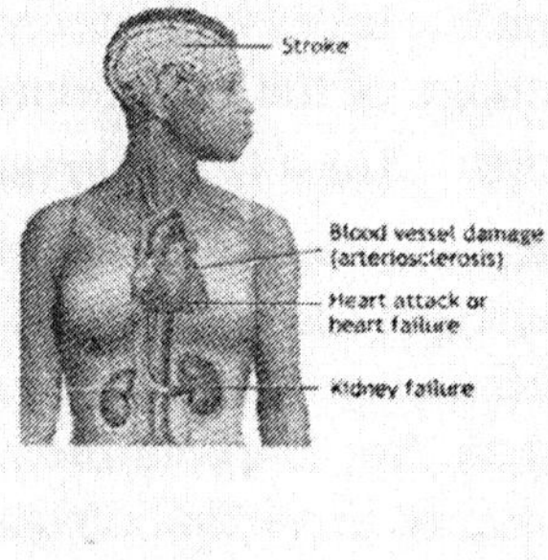

Q.95. What is CVA (cerebral vascular accident)?

Ans. CVA refers to sudden bursting of cerebral arteries, or embolism in the cerebral artery. This leads to non-supply of blood to the brain tissues, which are completely dependent on these arteries for blood.As a result, the nerves supply to that corresponding area of the body gets damaged or death of that area occurs. This leads to paralysis of one side of the body and this is often known as CVA (cerebral vascular accident).

Q.96. What is paralysis (stroke)?

Ans. Stroke is commonly known as paralysis. It is caused due to cerebral vascular accident. If the stoke occurs in the right side of the brain the left side of body usually gets paralyzed and vice-versa. This is called Hemiparesis or hemiplegia. The paraplegia is a stroke that occurs in the lower limbs. This condition is generally associated with high blood pressure. Because the blood becomes thick, the strokes are very common in coronary heart disease patients or those who are having blockages in the coronary arteries with high cholesterol and high triglycerides.

Q.97. How to reduce blood pressure?

Ans. It is necessary for a stroke patient, to control or to reduce the blood pressure to about 120/80 mmHg. If the blood pressure is not controlled it may prove fatal. Blood pressure can be reduced by changing life style, stress management, yoga, meditation and diet modification. Drugs for lowering the blood pressure are also available that can be given in the form of injections. The lowering of blood pressure will lead to a sudden improvement in stroke patients.

Q.98. What is the treatment of CVA?

Ans. Different types of CVA's have different types of treatments.

Q.99. What are the types of paralysis?

Ans. Monoplegia,Paraplegia,Hemiplegia,Hemiparesis.

Q.100. What is hemiplegia?

Ans. Hemiplegia refers to paralysis of one side of the body. It is the most common type of paralytic attack, in which one side of the body gets damaged or paralyzed, the nerves get affected, and the person cannot move either the right hand and the right leg or vice-versa. This is known as right hemiplegia. Right hemiplegia occurs when the stroke occurs in the left side of the brain that leads to paralysis of the right side of the body. Similarly, stroke on the right side of the brain leads to left hemiplegia. Individuals with paralytic attack do not die but their condition improves if proper care is given.

Q.101. What is paraplegia?

Ans. It is a type of paralysis in which clot or hemorrhage occurs in a particular part of the brain stem. As a result, the nerves supplying the lower part of the body get affected leading to paralysis of both the legs.

Q.102. What is Hemiparesis?

Ans. Hemiparesis is a mild form of stroke, where there is no complete paralysis but the muscles become weak. In this, one can move the hands and legs, but the power of the muscles is less. In such people there is no brain death so they show improvement. In these patients intra cranial pressure is raised and when it comes to normal they regain their power.

Q.103. What are the precautions to prevent CVA?

Ans. As person gets old, his blood pressure, cholesterol and triglycerides level increases, this increases the chances of Cerebro-Vascular Accident. Obesity and high level of stress also increase the chances of CVA. So care must be taken to keep the cholesterol and triglycerides level within the normal limits. Obesity must also be controlled and the level of stress should be reduced. If the blood pressure is very high, then it must be controlled by the use of drugs or by any other measure. If all this is properly followed, then the chances of developing hemiplegia, hemiperesis or CVA will be minimum. The people who are at risk of developing CVA are generally advised to take aspirin or any other blood thinning agents, to avoid embolus or hemorrhage. This can prevent stroke or paralysis and are very useful in preventing CVA.

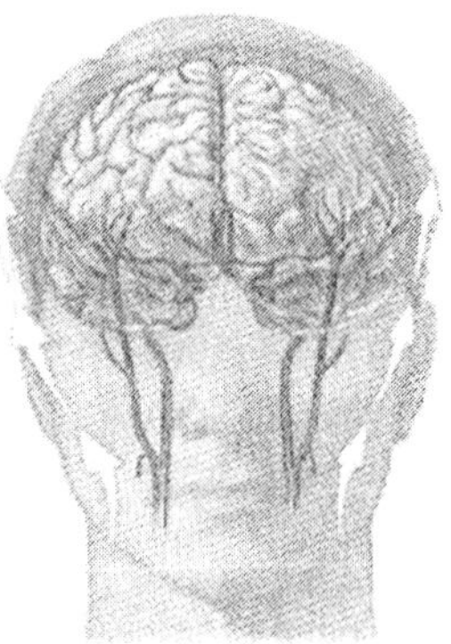

Q.104. What is Transient Ischaemic Attack (TIA)?

Ans. In Transient Ischemic Attack (TIA), due to high blood pressure, the spasm of the brain arteries or the cerebral arteries leads to sudden unconsciousness, for a few minutes. At this time the body may also get

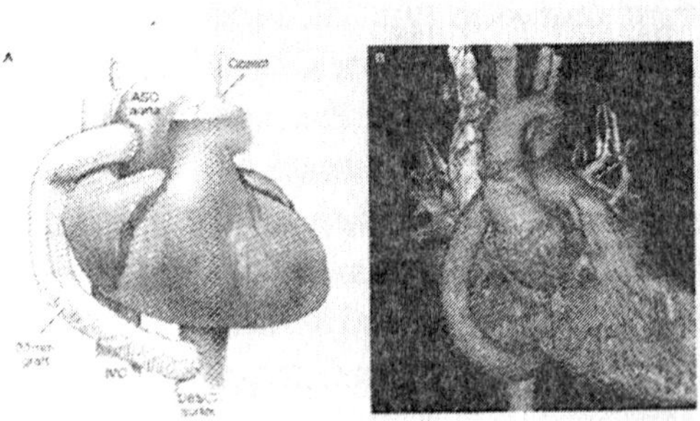

paralyzed for a minute. As soon as the recovery occurs the patient is saved from the heart attack. This is almost a pre-condition for a stroke. So the TIA gives an idea that there may be stroke in the future. If you have TIA, please be aware of this and immediately treat yourself by lowering blood pressure, cholesterol, cutting down fat, obesity and by controlling other factors.

8. HYPERTENSION IN YOUNG

Q.105. Why does hypertension occur in young?

Ans. Nowadays it is commonly seen that people as young as 15-20 years of age also develop high blood pressure. These people are generally obese; they eat lot of fried foods, live under stressful conditions and do very little physical work.

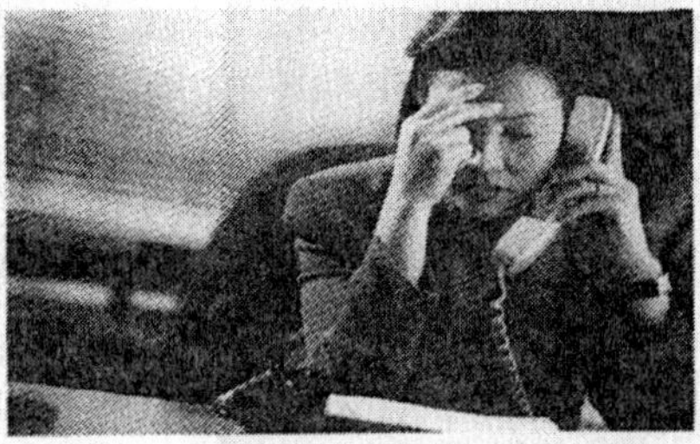

If blood pressure of a person above 15 years of age is more than 130/90 mmHg he is labeled as hypertensive.

Q.106. What are the causes of hypertension in young?

Ans. High blood pressure can be due to a number of factors. Some of these are listed as under:

- Obesity
- Eating fried food
- Excessive stress
- Heredity

Q.107. How can high blood pressure problem be solved in young people?

Ans. Nowadays blood pressure problem is increasing day by day in young people and it must be controlled immediately. Obese people are more prone to high blood pressure. They must take steps to reduce weight. Eat high fiber food and low fat food. Along with this they must also do meditation, yoga and go for walk regularly. This will help them to control their blood pressure. If the blood pressure is not controlled with any of the above measures then they must start taking medication to keep it within the normal limits.

Q.108. What should be the ideal blood pressure in young?

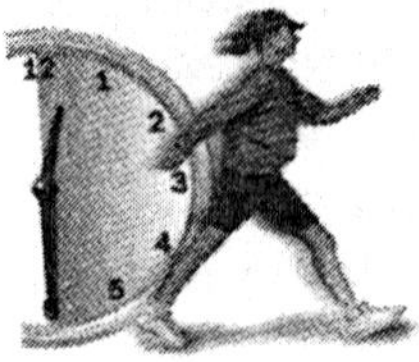

Ans. Till15 years of age the blood pressure of the young boys and girls should be lower than 120/80 mmHg. But after 15-16 years of age, their blood pressure should be 120/80mmHg. If their blood pressure is more than130mmHg, it is declared as hypertension in young.

Q.109. What are the complications of hypertension in young?

Ans. The complications of hypertension in young are: defect in vision, headache, restlessness, and anxiety. Some individuals may also get stroke due to the high blood pressure. Gastrointestinal problems are very common in hypertensive patients.

9. EXERCISE & HYPERTENSION:

Q.110. How does exercise help in reducing the blood pressure?

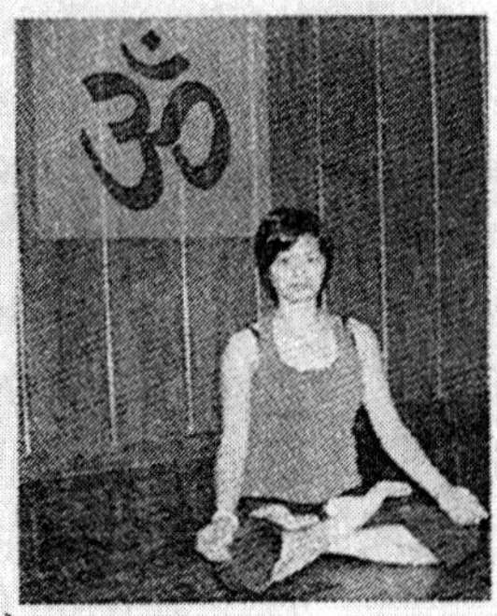

Ans. Regular exercise can help to reduce high blood pressure. This is because; exercise increases the vascular network inside the muscles. Also, the tubes inside the muscles can accommodate a lot of blood and there is ramping down of blood pressure. Such people, if they do exercise regularly their blood pressure can be controlled and their peripheral resistance also goes down.

Q111. What are the exercises for reducing the blood pressure?

Ans. Several exercises are helpful in reducing the blood pressure, but amongst all-walking is the best form of exercise.

Other flexible exercises like yoga and meditation are also helpful in reducing the weight and lowering the blood pressure.

Q.112. How much exercise should one do?

Ans. Regular exercise will control weight, and at the same time will help lower the blood pressure. A hypertensive patient can go for a brisk walk early in the morning for at least half an hour daily. They can also do skipping or spot jogging. If they want they can also join gym.

Q.113. Does yoga reduce the blood pressure?

Ans. Yes, yoga definitely reduces the blood pressure. It is not a simple exercise, but it has soothing effect on the brain. Yoga can cut down the stress and if the stress goes down then the blood pressure will immediately go down. There are many asanas for the hypertensive patients that can help them control their blood pressure. Sarwangasan, kayotsarg, health rejuvenating exercises are the major yoga asanas for the blood pressure patients.

Q.114. Does Pranayama reduce the blood pressure?

Ans. Doing pranayama regularly for 15-20 minutes can help in reducing the stress and strain, because it reduces the adrenaline level in the blood, which is very helpful in controlling blood pressure. Pranayama must be done empty stomach early morning. Anulom vilom pranayama is a best kind of pranayama, which a hypertension person must do. There are some other kinds of pranayama, which can increase the blood pressure. Therefore, Anulom vilom pranayama or Nadi-Shodhan pranayama must be practiced slowly and in a comfortable posture on a regular basis.

10. CAUSES OF HYPERTENSION:

Q.115. What are the causes of hypertension?

Ans. Hypertension is a very common diseases nowadays. This diseases can be due to a number of reasons, the most important being stress. It is seen that people who are more stressed usually have high blood pressure. The other factors that may also lead to hypertension include: obesity, wrong food habits, excessive salt intake and diabetes.

Q.116. Does stress lead to hypertension?

Ans. Yes, stress is the most important reason of hypertension. Anxiety, worry, anger and fear all increase the blood pressure. This is because during stress the heart rate increases, spasm of the arteries occurs and the blood pressure goes up.

Q.117. Does alcohol lead to hypertension?

Ans. Alcohol if taken in less amount acts as a vasodilator and does not lead to hypertension, but if it is taken in large amount it will ultimately increase the triglyceride level in blood, causing narrowing of the arteries, leading to hypertension. Also it is seen that alcohol consumption is more common in people who are living under stressful conditions.

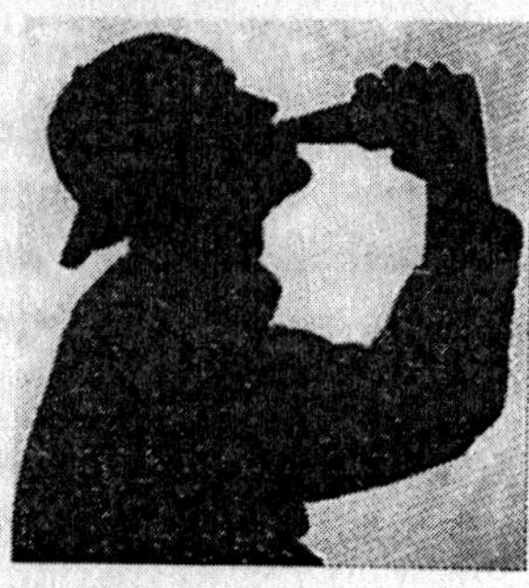

Q.118. Does smoking cause hypertension?

Ans. Smoking definitely causes hypertension. Smoking and hypertension usually co-exist. It is seen that people who smoke generally have high blood pressure. Smoking also helps to build up blockages in the arteries. This is because the internal membrane of a smoker becomes sticky due to deposition of nicotine. This favours the deposition of fat in the tubes leading to hypertension. Also smoking is more common in people who are living under stress, which in itself is a powerful risk factor of hypertension.

Q.119. Does irregular exercise lead to hypertension?

Ans. No, irregular exercise does not lead to hypertension. However a sedentary and stressful lifestyle may definitely lead to hypertension.

Q.120. Can hypertension occur due to poor food habits?

Ans. Yes, poor food habits may also lead to hypertension. Food is a very important aspect of our life. What and how much we eat directly influences our health and well-being. Excessive intake of fried foods, salt, low fiber and high calorie food increase the chances of hypertension. Irregular and unhygienic food habits may cause ill health, which can also lead to hypertension.

Q.121. Is heredity also a cause of hypertension?

Ans: For the vast majority of hypertensive patients, there is no one gene passed on (inherited) from patient to child that is responsible for high blood pressure. More likely, there are many different genes that interact with each other and the environment to produce high blood pressure. Therefore, inheritance predisposes a person to high blood pressure, but hypertension might only occur with the addition of one or more environmental factors.

11.STRESS AND HYPERTENSION:

Q.122. What are the causes of stress in our daily life?

Ans. In our daily life stress may occur due to a number of reasons. The most common cause of stress in our day-to-day life is imbalance between our income and expenditure. Our income remains the same but our wants (expenses) are unlimited. This breeds dissatisfaction leading to stress.

In the family, the number of family members have grown up, and every person in the family wants more and more facilities, somebody wants a car, somebody wants a mobile, some body wants a computer, somebody wants a scooter, a television, a fridge and so on. These desires lead people to take loans from banks, which causes stress. Inside the family people have become isolated, they have become self-centered, and people do not sacrifice for others. Another thing is that previously they used to stay together in the family and listen to others and would not protest. But nowadays people do not listen to any body, if you tell them that they are wrong, they immediately shout. This is one of the major reasons in the family. Along with these, there is pollution, there is traffic, there are rules and regulations, there are thieves and cheats all over, corruption is there, there are formalities like income tax, sales tax, duties, customs. All these ultimately lead to stress in our daily life, which gradually leads to hypertension.

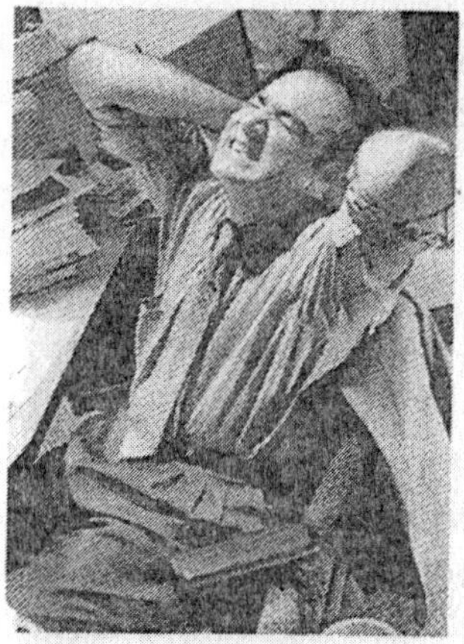

Q.123. How does stress cause hypertension?

Ans. Stress or the psychological pressure or emotional dissatisfaction releases some chemicals in the body, known as catacolamines. Adrenaline is one of the catacolamine, which is secreted more when we are under stress. Adrenaline causes spasm in the arteries (narrowing of the arteries) all over the body, increases the heart rate and simultaneously the blood pressure rises.

Q.124. What happens in stress?

Ans. In stress, certain changes occur in our body like:-

1. Increase in heart rate.
2. Increase in blood pressure
3. Rise in blood sugar
4. Gastritis, paralysis, stroke and heart problems may also occur because stress increases the cholesterol level in the blood.

Q.125 How is stress reduced?

Ans. Stress can be reduced in three steps:-

1. Do not produce stress.
2. If there is stress, then try to release it as soon as possible.

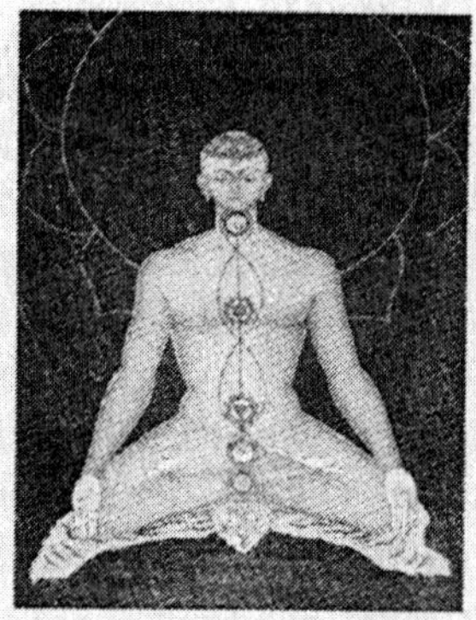

3. Manage the stress on your own, because in daily life, stress is often produced by ourselves. If one can manage stress, then the stress can be reduced. Stress can never be zero or nil, but if one cuts down the stress by 50% it can help to reduce the blood pressure.

Another way of reducing stress is by training the cerebral cortex or the logical brain, which stores information about the things going around us. If the logical brain is trained about the wrong things happening in India, then the stress can be cut down to some extent. There is another part of brain, which is known as emotional brain or the limbic cortex or the illogical brain. Whenever something goes against us, the illogical brain disturbs the body functions and increases the blood pressure.

Q.126. How to know if the blood pressure is due to stress?

Ans. Stress and hypertension are closely related to each other. To find out if the blood pressure is due to stress or do not measure the blood pressure of the patient and find the reading on the upper side. Now make the patient to relax by putting him in savasana, the blood pressure immediately goes down. Another way of finding out is to check the blood pressure in the morning after getting up from the bed and then again in the evening. If your blood pressure is high it means that it is due to stress.

Q.127. How does yoga help in stress reduction?

Ans. Yoga is a kind of stretching exercise in which all the muscles of the body get stretched, and thus they get relaxed. When one does yoga asanas the brain also relaxes.

The Yoga has two components: YAMA and NIYAMA. These two components are very effective in stress management. YAMA is the asana, which people should not do and the NIYAMA is the asana, which people should do.

Along with yoga, pranayam and meditation also help in reducing the blood pressure. Nowadays, research has shown that meditation helps in reducing the blood pressure much faster than medicines.

Q128. How does meditation help to reduce stress?

Ans. Preksha Dhyan is an advanced type of meditation. In this along with stress reduction relaxation of body also occurs. It is usually practiced in a comfortable sitting position.

A famous Jain saint "Acharya Shri Tulshi" and his successor "Yuya Acharya" who is now leading the preksha dhyan meditation have propagated Preksha Dhyan system. Along with Jain saint, other people who have learnt prekshadhyan are also spreading this system.

Q.129. What is kayotsarg?

Ans. Kayotsarg is a kind of relaxation technique. It is also a type of meditation that is very easy to practice. In kayotsarg the whole body is relaxed. It is also termed as progressive relaxation. When you lay down you relax. But in kayotsarg you progressively relax. That means your body will gradually get relaxed, relaxed... and relaxed.

To do kayotsarg, one has to choose a room in which there is no sound and the temperature is also very stable. In this one has to lie down on the bed or on a carpet and think about every part of the body that it is getting relaxed. This helps to decrease the stress and reduce blood pressure. Kayotsarg is very helpful for people with stress related high blood pressure.

Q.130. How can stress be managed?

Ans. Stress can be managed in three ways: -

1. By not producing stress.
2. Cutting down stress
3. Stress Management.

Managing stress is based upon understanding the cause of stress and relaxing oneself.

For this, one has to understand the processes i.e. Anekant which means that for one thing there may be several opinions, and if one does not argue and agrees with others then he can cut down on stress.

Another way of managing stress is to go to the root of the stress.

Communicating and sharing views with others is also a part of stress management, because if one does not share their views it can also increase the blood pressure.

Q.131. How much stress do I have?

Ans. Stress cannot be measured in any unit. Close observation of the daily activities of the person shows if he is under stress or not. For example: while driving a car if the driver shouts on another this indicates that he is under stress.

Q.132. What is subconscious stress?

Ans. During sleep if a person dreams about bad things, which are due to stress, then it is termed as subconscious stress.

Q.133. How to know if I am under stress?

Ans. Stress can be identified by physical symptoms like:

1. Sweating palms
2. Cold fingers
3. Dry mouth
4. Shaky hands
5. Frequent urination
6. Diarrhoea
7. Change of tone of speech
8. Nausea
9. Restlessness

Q.134. How much time should I spend on meditation or kayotsarg?

Ans. Meditation or Kayotsarg is a very good exercise for relaxing our body. These exercises chain our emotional brain or the limbic cortex. In other words, they relax the limbic system of the brain. It is the site of all our emotions, irritability, and jealousy. So, by doing meditation or kayotsarg stress can be reduced. 10-15minutes of meditation must be practiced daily.

Q.135. Can stress management cure hypertension?

Ans. Yes, definitely 90% cases of hypertension can be cured to a great extent by managing stress. Stress is the major factor, which leads to hypertension. It can also be cured by weight reduction, cessation of smoking and cutting down salt in the food.

There are many people who live their life comfortably with normal blood pressure but whenever some dispute occurs, the blood pressure immediately shoots up. So, by controlling stress blood pressure can be controlled.

Q.136. Why do people fight?

Ans. Fight is an expression of stress. Everyone has his or her own way of thinking. Whenever views of two people clash fighting results.

For example, if husband and wife have different viewpoints and they do not agree with each other's view, then there will be clashes. In other words, if we do not get what we want fight may occur. To avoid this, one has to understand the other person's mind. This is called Anekant. Anekant means every person has different opinion. One must accept this and show respect towards the other person's view and should not fight.

Q.137. How can financial stress be managed?

Ans. Money plays an important role in everyone's life. For example- for every want or activity one needs money. So balancing the money sector is very important. Nowadays, most of the people are stressed due to financial problem. This is because they spend more than their income. But if they could manage to control expenditure or if their expenditure is less than their income, the financial stress will immediately disappear. But if their expenditure increases than their income, the stress will also increase. To reduce stress, it is necessary to strike a balance between income and expenditure.

Saving is another way of managing stress. If one saves a small percent of this income; it will help him in case of need. Thus, saving also helps to reduce financial stress in emergency situations.

Q.138. Do satsangs help to reduce stress?

Ans. Yes. Our subconscious mind is full of good things. By visiting satsang you may continuously remember what things are good or how to behave. Such satsangs are beneficial, if one hears everyday, and tries to apply them in your daily life, to live a peaceful and happy life, we need lot of advice which we already know. But in satsang, when we hear them again and again, it changes our mind and helps to apply them in our life.

Q.139. How can we control Ego?

Ans. Ego makes people feel, that they are good or superior to others. This leads to a lot of stress, if they fail to prove their superiority. So, to reduce ego a person should try to find out his bad qualities and other people's good qualities. But if you see the bad qualities of others, then you feel yourself superior. And if you feel the good qualities of other, then you can understand that your ego is not justified. So, to cut down ego you have to understand a term known as Harmony- in Hindi it means Har—mani. If you understand your own fault and know that you cannot be the best in all fields, then your ego will definitely come down.

Q.140. How to speak so that it does not cause stress?

Ans. Communication is a very effective way of expressing one's feelings. It has been seen, that lot of people have wrong way of communication or speaking and this often leads to stress. On the other hand, some people speak in such a way, that it does not cause stress and your message is conveyed. This is called the good way of speaking, one should always communicate in such a way, that it should not make the other person embrace or their feeling should hurt. For example– If you do not like some body work, then instead of saying that I am not happy with your work and I feel you should do like this, but you are saying that you are an idiot, you do not know how to do it. Then you are insulting the other person. So, please do not insult any body, always speak in good and polite manner.

Q.141. Why blood pressure rises when going for an interview or an exam?

Ans: The common cause of hypertension is stress. During examination or at the time of an interview there is tremendous stress, due to more secretion of a hormone called adrenaline. This hormone increases the flow of blood and the heart rate, which leads to high blood pressure.

12. MISCELLANEOUS

Q.142. What is the blood pressure in lungs?

Ans. In a normal subject with minimal pulmonary valve regurgitation. Diastolic gradient= 3.9 mmHg

Assuming normal (= 6 mmHg) right atrial pressure, wedge pressure= 3.9+6= 9.9 mmHg.

Estimated increased wedge pressure.

Continuous wave Doppler tracing, transthoracic examination.

Patient with minimal pulmonary valve regurgitation.

Diastolic gradient= 15.2 mmHg

Assuming normal (= 6 mmHg) right atrial pressure, wedge pressure= 15.2+6= 21.2mmHg.

Q.143. What is pulmonary hypertension?

Ans. Pulmonary hypertension is a disorder of the blood vessels in the lungs. "Pulmonary" means "in the lungs," and "hypertension" means "high blood pressure."

Pulmonary hypertension happens when the blood pressure in the pulmonary arteries (the vessels that carry blood from the heart to the lungs) becomes higher than normal. This puts strain on the right side of the heart.

Q.144. What are the symptoms of pulmonary hypertension?

Ans. Common signs of pulmonary hypertension are shortness of breath with activity, feeling tired, fainting and chest pain. Symptoms usually limit the exercise and other activities.

Q.145. What are the causes of pulmonary hypertension?

Ans. Pulmonary hypertension can be due to a number of reasons. Sometimes the cause is not known. When the cause of pulmonary hypertension is not known, the disorder is called "primary" pulmonary hypertension.

"Secondary" pulmonary hypertension has a known cause. Common causes are emphysema and chronic bronchitis (breathing problems). Other causes are congestive heart failure, birth defects in the heart, chronic pulmonary thrombo-embolism (old blood clots in the pulmonary arteries), HIV infection (AIDS), and certain medicines, including the diet drugs fenfluramine and dexfenfluramine. (These diet drugs are no longer available.)

Both primary and secondary types are usually permanent conditions, although treatment can improve symptoms and long-term outcomes in some people.

Q.146. What is the treatment of pulmonary hypertension?

Ans. Pulmonary hypertension usually needs separate treatment. It is a serious illness, but treatment is possible. One may be treated with oxygen, agents to help your heart pump well, diuretics, anticoagulants (blood thinners), and medications to lower your pulmonary hypertension. Sometimes lung transplants also need to be done.

Q.147. Can blood pressure differ if measured in both arms?

Ans. Yes, it will be different in both arms. In the right hand the blood pressure will be more than the left hand. But this difference is not more than 5-6mmHg; this is because the right hand gets the blood supply first, from the heart than the left hand.

Q.148. Can blood pressure be measured in legs?

Ans: Yes, blood pressure can also be measured in legs. When the blood pressure is very low or the brachial arteries present in the hand are not palpable due to some reason, then the blood pressure can be measured in the legs. The same sound can be heard in the femoral artery present in the legs.

Q.149. Does the blood pressure differ in the upper arms and legs?

Ans. Yes, the blood pressure differs in upper arms and legs. The normal blood pressure in legs is 90% of the upper arm pressure, but it will be less if there is narrowing of the leg arteries.

Q.150. If the person is grossly obese then how to measure the blood pressure?

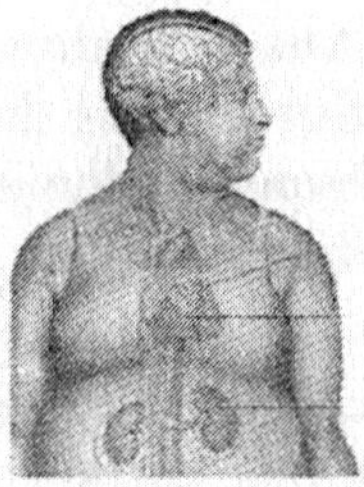

Ans. For the obese person, there is a special type of cuff available in the market, which is bigger in size than the normal cuff. This cuff can be easily wrapped round the upper arm of the grossly obese patient. We can also measure the blood pressure on ankle of the obese patient.

Q.151. What is the normal blood pressure in children?

Ans. Blood pressure in children differs with age. If the child's age is around three years, then his normal blood pressure is above107/69mmHg, at the age of ten the blood pressure should be above 117/75mmHg.

Q.152. Does obesity lead to hypertension?

Ans. Yes, obesity has been associated with hypertension. Hypertension may be affected by both build as well as by fatness. Weight reduction has been associated with a decrease in blood pressure in obese people. It has been proved that blood pressure rises according to the level of weight gain.

13.HEART AND ITS FUNCTIONS

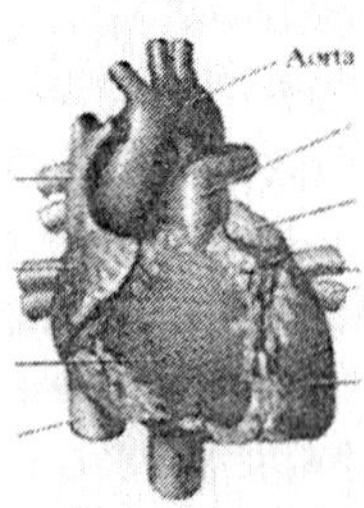

Q.153. What are the functions of the heart?

Ans. The function of heart is to pump the blood to the whole body. Heart beats 72 times per minute. It has four chambers. The chambers 1 and 3 pump first, so that the blood can be pushed from 1 - 2 and 3 –4.

After this, the chambers 2 and 4 pump together. From chamber 2 the blood goes to the lungs, where it mixes with oxygen and goes to chamber 3. From there the blood goes to chamber 4 and from chamber 4 the blood passes to the whole body.

After the body has used up all the oxygen present in the blood, the impure blood comes back to the chamber 1.This process goes on continuously in the body, and is known as circulation process.

Q.154. How is heart responsible for increasing the blood pressure?

Ans. Heart pumps the blood to the whole body. If the blood pressure is normal the heart also works normally. But if the heart rate goes up like in the case of excitement, the blood pressure rises. In excitement the heart's pumping power increases. It contracts more forcefully, increasing the blood pressure. Some chemicals are also released inside the body called adrenaline, angiotensin, which increases the blood pressure through the heart.

Q.155. How does high blood pressure affect the heart?

Ans. Blood pressure also affects the heart. The chamber no. 4 or the left ventricle of the heart pumps out the blood, at a pressure of 120mmHg. But if due to some reason the pumping power of the heart is increased, the blood pressure also increases. For example, if the blood pressure is 150-160mmHg then the heart has to pump the blood more forcefully and fastly, to continue the circulation process.

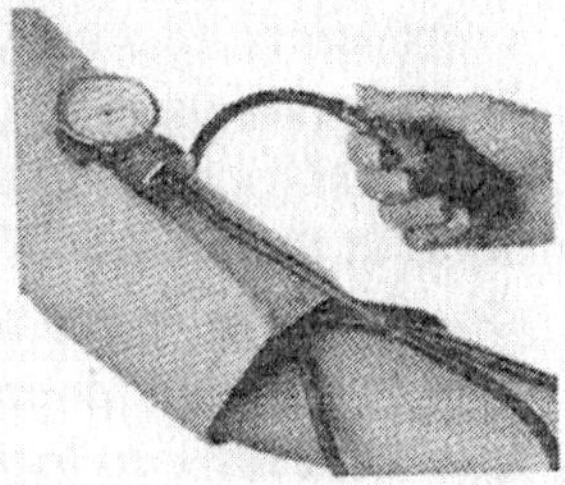

If high blood pressure persists for a long time, the heart muscles become thick. This is known as LVH (left ventricular hypertrophy). Due to LVH, the heart needs more blood, and this may lead to angina. Usually at the time of heart attack, the blood pressure is very high. The heart cannot pump blood very well and water gets deposited inside the lungs, which leads to breathlessness. This is known as heart failure or LVF (left ventricular failure).

14. LOW BLOOD PRESSURE

Q.156. What is low blood pressure/hypotension?

Ans. Our normal blood pressure is about 120/80mmHg. When the systolic blood pressure is below 100mmHg and diastolic is less than 70mmHg then it is known as low blood pressure or hypotension.

Q.157. How to identify low blood pressure?

Ans. In low blood pressure, the patient feels giddiness especially in standing position. This is because the brain, which is the upper most part of the body, does not get enough blood. He also complains of weakness. The person may also have sweating, he feels less energetic, and gets tired easily.

Q.158. What are the causes of low blood pressure?

Ans. Most of the people with low blood pressure do not have any symptoms. Low blood pressure occurs due to vitamin deficiency, wrong food habits, and loss of fluid from the body due to diarrhoea etc.

Q.159. What is an ideal blood pressure?

Ans. Our ideal blood pressure is 120/80mmHg. However, according to a new research the ideal blood pressure should be about 115/75mmHg.

Q.160. How can low BP be treated?

Ans. In many cases, low blood pressure may not need any treatment because the person, who has low blood pressure, does not have any complaints. In such cases no treatment is required, only when the low blood pressure gives symptoms then it needs treatment. If a person has normal blood pressure and it suddenly falls down, then it is required to look at the causes of low blood pressure, that whether it is because of diarrhoea, or if the person is not taking adequate fluid. It can also be due to fever, or anemia that the blood pressure can go down. In such cases we have to look for the causes and treat it.

And if there is low blood pressure for a certain time, then it is good to give a lot of salt in the person's food, or to give a cup of coffee/tea which stimulates the heartbeat and so the blood pressure goes up.

If there is a severe low blood pressure, then the person is injected with a normal saline in the form of drip, and this is a very common treatment in the hospital, when the patient reaches there with a low blood pressure.

Other case can be, if there is a hemorrhage or bleeding inside the body, the blood pressure suddenly goes down. In such cases blood may be transfered.

Q.161. What to do if the blood pressure falls suddenly?

Ans. Whenever the blood pressure falls suddenly, we have to look at the cause that whether it is because of accident leading to internal hemorrhage or from outside if some artery is cut or some bleeding is occurring, it can also be due to dehydration, if fluid is not taken in adequate amount. In such cases the treatment according to the cause should be given immediately, to increase the blood pressure.

15. RENAL HYPERTENSION

Q.162. What is renal hypertension or renovascular hypertension?

Ans. The arteries that carry blood to the kidneys get narrowed due to the deposition of cholesterol and triglycerides. Due to these blockages, the blood pressure increases in kidney. This is known as renal hypertension or reno-vascular hypertension

Q.163. What are the causes of renal hypertension?

Ans. Blood pressure is determined by the amount of blood pumped by the heart, and the size and condition of the arteries. Several other factors can affect blood pressure including the volume of water in the body, salt content of the body; condition of the kidneys, nervous system, or blood vessels, and levels of various hormones in the body.

Renovascular hypertension, is a form of secondary hypertension (hypertension caused by another condition in the body). It occurs in less than 5% of all people with hypertension. Symptoms usually begin before the age of 30years or after 50years of age, depending on the cause of the damage to the kidney blood vessels. Narrowing of the renal artery reduces blood flow to the kidneys. Stenosis is often related to atherosclerosis, but may be caused by injury to the artery that causes scarring. Reduced blood flow to the kidney, leads to an excessive release of the hormone renin, a potent hormone that increases blood pressure.

Q.164. What are the symptoms of renal hypertension?

Ans. Headache is an occasional symptom. If the hypertension is severe, symptoms may include:

- Tiredness
- Confusion
- Vision changes
- Nausea and vomiting
- Angina-like chest pain (crushing chest pain)
- Congestive heart failure

Q.165. How does high blood pressure affect the kidneys?

Ans. Kidneys are affected because the arteries (renal arteries) which supply blood to the kidney become narrow, due to an increase in the blood pressure and this does not allow the blood to flow smoothly to the kidneys. This affects the normal function of kidneys. If it is prolonged, a complete blockage of blood flow to the kidney often results in permanent kidney failure.

Q.166. What diet should be given to a renal hypertension patient?

Ans: Renal hypertension patient should be given a low protein diet. This is because in a renal patient, urea gets accumulated and it is not excreted out in the urine. In such case low quality protein foods like dals, bread, and vegetables should be restricted. However, high quality protein foods like milk, cheese can be given in a very small amount. Secondly, due to high blood pressure sodium (salt) restriction also becomes necessary. Phosphorus, which is a mineral, should also be restricted in these patients because it is rich in protein.

Q.167. At what age does renal hypertension mostly occur?

Ans. Renal hypertension generally occurs before 30 years of age or after 50 years, depending upon the cause of the damage to the kidney blood vessels. Reno vascular hypertension is a form of secondary hypertension (hypertension caused by another condition in the body). It occurs in less than 5% of hypertensive population.

Q.168. Who can suffer from renal hypertension?

Ans. Patient with high blood pressure, high cholesterol, triglycerides and low HDL can suffer from renal hypertension. Also the people who smoke, consume alcohol, those who are obese are at high risk of renal hypertension.

Q.169. Does obesity affect renal hypertension?

Ans. Yes, obesity is also a risk factor for renal hypertension. In obese individuals the cholesterol and triglyceride levels are usually high, which leads to the blockages in the renal arteries and thus the blood pressure increases. So, patients with renal hypertension must reduce their weight by doing regular exercise and by taking low calorie diet.

Q.170. What is the treatment of renal hypertension?

Ans. The aim of treatment is to control the blood pressure. Medications that may be used in an attempt to control blood pressure include diuretics, beta-blockers, calcium channel blockers, angiotensin-converting enzyme inhibitors, angiotensin receptor blockers (ARBs) and alpha-blockers. Diazoxide or nitroprusside may be given in the hospital if symptoms are acute. Response to medications is highly individual. Blood pressure should be monitored frequently. Medication and dosage may need frequent adjustment.

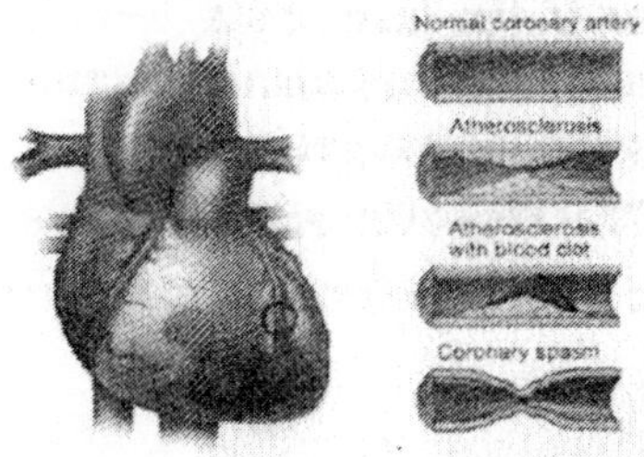

Surgical reconstruction of a damaged artery may also be performed. Balloon angioplasty or stenting of the damaged artery, may be used instead of open reconstruction.

Lifestyle changes are recommended, including weight loss, exercise, and dietary adjustments. Stop smoking and drinking alcohol. These habits add to the effects of hypertension.

16. COMPLICATIONS OF HYPERTENSION

Q.171. What are the complications of hypertension?

Ans: The major complications of hypertension are:

(a) Coronary artery disease and congestive heart failure
(b) Renal Failure
(c) Stroke
(d) Atherosclerosis
(e) Retinopathy

Q.172. How does hypertension affect the heart?

Ans: Hypertension plays a significant role in the development of arteriosclerosis and atherosclerosis (blockages). Hypertension reduces the elasticity of vessels, allowing cholesterol and triglycerides to deposit in the form of atheromas, which in turn lead to thrombus formation and possible emboli formation. This disturbs the blood flow and leads to ischemic disease.

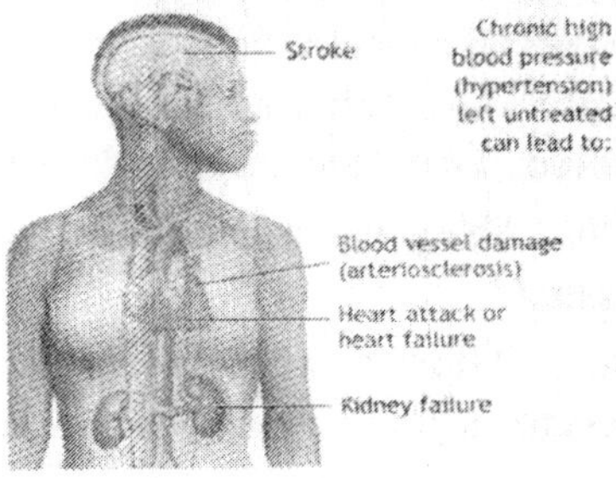

Coronary heart disease is the leading cause of death in hypertensive patients. Ventricular hypertrophy occurs as a result of increased cardiac output in the face of systemic vascular resistance. Eventually, the heart is unable to maintain this constant output and the hypertrophied muscle outstrips its oxygen supply.

Q.173. How does hypertension affect the brain?

Ans: High blood pressure can affect the brain in many ways. It can accelerate the effects of atherosclerosis, a condition characterized by narrowing of the arteries due to the build-up of fatty plaques. It can also break the blockages and release cholesterol plaques from the artery walls, which can then block blood flow to the brain (embolic stroke), weaken artery walls, leading to vessel breakage and bleeding into the brain hemorrhagic stroke), thicken the artery walls due to the constant stress load. It can also cause a hemorrhagic stroke in people born with rare malformations of the blood vessels in the brain.

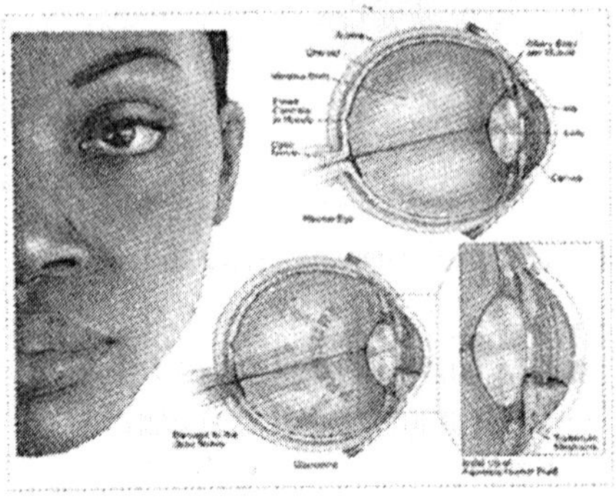

Q.174. How does hypertension affect the eyes?

Ans. Due to high blood pressure, the arteries of the eyes that are not supported by side arteries get damaged. When the blood pressure is very high there is some exudation in the retina. It means, the fluid is leaking inside the retina and this part of the retina gets damaged. Loss of vision occurs, when the pressure increases in the retina, which can be diagnosed by an ophthalmoscope.

Q.175. Why do patients with hypertension get a cardiac arrest?

Ans. Coronary artery disease (CAD) patients with hypertension often get cardiac arrest because the internal membrane which guards the blockage to fall into the blood, becomes thinner and thinner due to the deposition of more fats, and with high blood pressure they easily get ruptured and form a clot in the artery, it means the artery gets 100% blocked. This is known as heart attack or cardiac arrest.

Q.176. Why is it necessary to control the blood pressure before a surgery?

Ans. There are many superficial arteries present in the body. If the pressure is high and cut is made, massive bleeding will occur. In such cases the patient may also die. So, before surgery it is necessary to maintain the blood pressure within the normal range. Even an anesthetic refuses to give anesthesia if the blood pressure of the patient is high.

17. WOMEN AND HYPERTENSION

Q.177. What is the normal blood pressure for women?

Ans. Scientifically, the blood pressure in both men and women are almost same. There is no distinction done in the recommendation. But it is usually seen that women have lower blood pressure than men. In India, the blood pressure of women is normally 110/70mmHg.Although the reason is not known, but it may be due to continuous loss of blood in the form of menstrual period and anaemia which can lead to low blood pressure.

And the other reason may be that in our societies women do not have too much work pressure or pressure of money earning like men do.

Q.178. Why high blood pressure occurs in women?

Ans. Nowadays high blood pressure is very common in women. This is mainly due to the increasing level of stress in their lives. Previously women did not work so hard. They had to take care of their household chores and these were not very difficult, everything was stereotype. There was no work pressure. They would get lot of time to rest. But in this modern world both husband and wife work outside the home. Women have to do the double job as a housewife compared to a workingwomen, and also there is pressure from everywhere to perform well.

Many women are overweight. They consume very high fatty food. This could be the other reason, that nowadays blood pressure is high in women.

Q179. What is pre delivery hypertension?

Ans. Before delivery, there is secretion of bad hormones in women's body. This is known as toxemia (pre eclampsia) that raises the blood pressure, and protein in the urine. Women with pre-eclampsia generally have symptoms like swelling in hands and feet, fever, headache, overweight, dizziness and intense stomach pain. It is also known as PIH (pregnancy induced hypertension)

Q.180. What is post delivery hypertension?

Ans. High blood pressure in pregnancy may occur due to a condition unrelated to pregnancy (such as essential hypertension or secondary hypertension) that begins or continues during pregnancy. The rise in blood pressure may have preceeded the pregnancy by months or years. However, this rise is first noticed during pregnancy. This is known as post delivery hypertension or chronic hypertension, which continues after the baby is delivered. Women with chronic hypertension are at an increased risk of developing pre-eclampsia.

Q.181. Should we use medicine to control Pre-delivery hypertension?

Ans. Yes, if the hypertension is not controlled in pregnancy induced or in pre delivery stage, then the medications must be started. High blood pressure may also damage the fetus or an abortion may occur. Excessive bleeding may also occur. Therefore, medicines must be used to control pre delivery hypertension.

Q.182. What happens to this kind of hypertension after delivery?

Ans. Usually at the time of delivery, the blood pressure returns to normal. In such cases, one has to look at the causes and try to solve them, like to reduce weight, to reduce the stress by which the blood pressure can be lowered down.

Q.183. Does diet control give some relief in post delivery hypertension?

Ans. Yes, diet control, regular exercise and stress management can improve the post delivery blood pressure.

Q.184. Do oral contraceptive pills increase the blood pressure?

Ans. Oral contraceptive pills are very commonly used to control the birth rate. These medicines contain small amount of estrogen and progesterone hormones that prevent pregnancy. But earlier these pills used to contain large amount of these hormones, which increases the blood pressure. Nowadays they contain a small amount of these hormones, which increase the systolic blood pressure to a very small degree. If the blood pressure is increasing by taking contraceptives, then one should avoid taking these pills for some time and the blood pressure will come down.

Q.185. Does menopause affect hypertension in women?

Ans. Progesterone and estrogen hormones in women help to control the blood pressure. After menopause these hormones are not secreted, which may lead to an increase in the blood pressure thereby increasing the risk of cardiovascular disease. Hormone replacement therapy is usually advised to menopausal women to decrease the risk of hypertension and cardiovascular disease.

18. ALTERNATIVE THERAPIES AND HYPERTENSION CONTROL

Q.186. What is the alternative treatment for hypertension?

Ans. For a hypertension patient besides medication, other alternative treatments are also available. For example, imparting knowledge about food will help a hypertensive make intelligent food choices and thus help him control blood pressure more effectively.

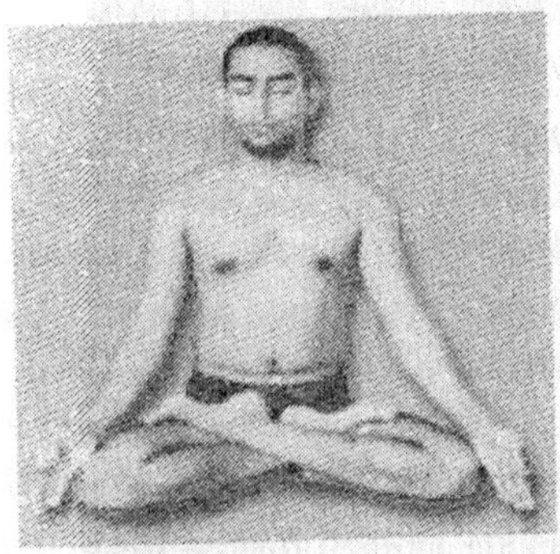

Hypertension can also be controlled by exercise, yoga, stress management and walking. Since obesity is one of the risk factors for hypertension, weight reduction also helps hypertensives.

Q.187. Does yoga help to control hypertension?

Ans. Yes, it helps to control hypertension. Yoga is usually advocated for mental relaxation as it helps in improving personal response to the environment. There are various asanas, which helps in normalizing blood pressure. The most effective asanas are:

(1) Yama **(2) Niyam**

These two are basically used for stress management, because as you know by controlling stress, hypertension can also be ultimately controlled.

Q.188. Does regular exercise control hypertension?

Ans. Regular exercise can help to control hypertension to a great extent. Stressful and sedentary lifestyle with lack of exercise, leads to obesity, which is a risk factor for hypertension. By doing regular exercise, weight can be reduced and this results in the lowering of blood pressure. Hypertensive patients should avoid strenuous exercises and should go for brisk walk early morning.

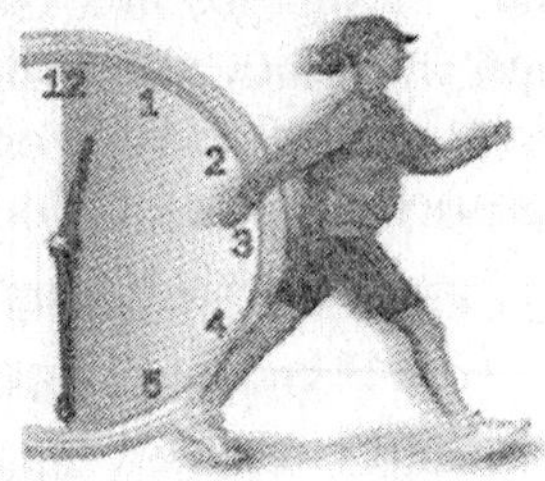

Q.189. Does regular walking help to control hypertension?

Ans. Going for a regular brisk walk will definitely control the hypertension because it helps to reduce the weight. Reduction of weight simultaneously results in lowering of blood pressure.

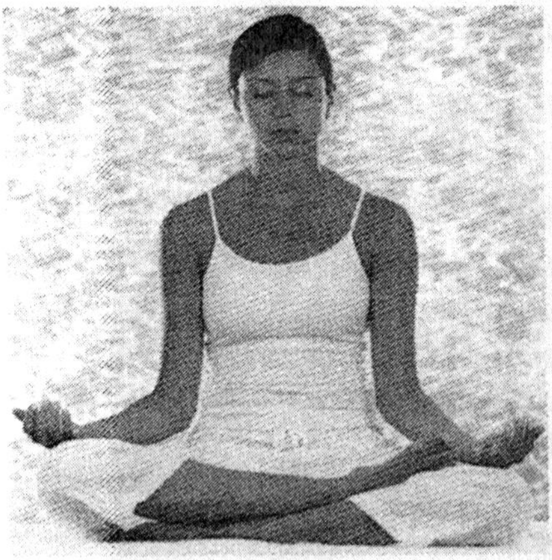

Q.190. Does meditation help to control hypertension?

Ans. Yes, meditation helps to control hypertension because meditation can reduce a variety of problems, that affects people mentally and emotionally and by which stress can cause and lead to hypertension. So, by doing meditation, all the stress can be cut down and by which blood pressure can ultimately be reduced. The constant chanting of a silently repeated word like mantra helps to achieve relaxation by avoiding external thoughts.

Q.191 Does kayotsarg help to control hypertension?

Ans. Kayotsarg is a kind of relaxation method. It is a type of meditation but it is easy to do. It is definitely useful in controlling BP.

In Kayatsarg, relaxation of the whole body occurs in a lying down position. For this, quite and comfortable environment is required. Alongwith relaxation, self awareness too is an implication of kayotsarga.

19. DIABETES MELLUTUS & HYPERTENSION

Q.192. What is diabetes?

Ans. Diabetes is a condition in which the glucose (sugar) level in blood increases above the normal limits. This condition develops due to lack or inefficiency of insulin, a hormone produced in the pancreas. The normal limit of blood sugar is:-

Fasting: 70-100 mg/dl

Post Prandial (2 hours after meal): 100 to 140 mg/dl

Random: < 140 mg/dl

To label a person as diabetic one reading is not sufficient. One must get at least three readings and all three must come positive.

Q.193. What are the symptoms of diabetes?

Ans. Diabetes is a disease which may remain asymptomatic for a long period of time before getting detected. A disease known to cause a number of complications involving almost all the organs of the body, this disease commonly gets detected on routine examination or when the patient reports with one of its complications.

The classical symptoms of diabetes are the three P's i.e. polyuria (increased urination), polydipsia (increased thirst) and polyphagia (increased hunger), combined with loss of weight. People with diabetes usually complain of non-healing of their wounds. They also suffer from frequent infections. Due to more urination there is loss of water leading to excessive thirst known as polydypsia. Excess urination also results in weight loss because of the glucose lost in the urine. There is fatigue, muscular weakness and the person feels lethargic. There may also be impotence.

In certain diabetics, white spots may be seen on the shoes after urination. In the advanced phase of diabetes some people face complications like kidney failure, loss of sensations (neuropathy) and blurred vision (retinopathy).

Q.194. What is the normal sugar level in blood?

Ans. Our normal fasting blood sugar is70-100 mg%. Everyone should try to keep the blood sugar within this range. Blood sugar is properly tested when a person fasts for 12 hours. At this time blood sugar remains in a normal state that our basal body will get.

Blood sugar that is measured at anytime during the day, when some amount of food is taken in the last 12 hours, it is known as random blood sugar and the one that is measured after two hour of meal is known as postprandial blood sugar. This should not be more than 140 mg%.

Q.195. How does diabetes mellitus lead to Hypertension?

Ans. There is no direct connection between hypertension and diabetes. It is commonly seen, many hypertensive people have diabetes also or vice versa. The real cause is not known, but there is a possibility that in diabetes the heart arteries get damaged and this may lead to high blood pressure.

Q.196. Why do diabetes mellitus patients usually become hypertensive?

Ans. The real cause is not known but it is true that diabetic patients usually get hypertension. Besides this obesity, lack of activity and stress lead to both diabetes and hypertension.

Q.197. What diet should be given to a patient with diabetes mellitus and high blood pressure?

Ans There are many food restrictions for a diabetic hypertensive patient. A diabetic hypertensive patient should avoid simple carbohydrates like rice, potato, sugar and sweet fruits like grapes, cheeku, mango and banana. Being a hypertensive he must also restrict salt in the diet and avoid high fat food.

Q.198. Can exercise help to reduce the hypertension in the diabetic patients?

Ans. If a hypertensive person also suffers from diabetes mellitus then he must do regular exercise. These two diseases are usually seen in obese individuals. Regular exercise not only helps in weight reduction but it also helps to reduce the blood sugar and the blood pressure.

Q.199. Can yoga help to reduce hypertension in diabetic patients?

Ans. Yes, yoga helps to reduce the high blood pressure and sugar levels of diabetic patients. Many types of asanas, help in reducing the blood pressure and blood sugar. One of the asanas that helps to reduce the sugar level is Ardhamatshyendrasana. This asana is considered especially good for diabetic patients. In this, there is complete twist of the abdomen region. This results in the squeezing of pancreas leading to an increased secretion of insulin, that helps to utilize the glucose more effectively, thereby lowering the blood sugar. Yoga asanas are also beneficial in lowering down the blood pressure. This is because hypertension mostly occurs in obese people. Regularly practicing yoga helps to cut down the extra weight, which also lowers the blood pressure.

Q. 200. How is hypertension controlled in a diabetic patient?

Ans. Blood pressure in a diabetic patient can be controlled by reducing the stress, reducing the weight, by doing regular yoga and exercise, along with this diabetic patient must have to make restrictions in their diet. They should avoid salt, sugar and simple carbohydrates.

Along with this high blood pressure medicine and high blood sugar medicine are to be continued to control the hypertension and sugar problem.

Q.201. What are the medicines to be used in patients with high blood pressure and high blood sugar?

Ans. Hypertensive & diabetic patients are usually treated with ACE-Inhibitors. Along with this modifications in diet and lifestyle can prove to be of great importance to such patients. Examples of ACE Inhibitots are listed in the chapter on **MEDICINES FOR TREATMENT OF HIGH BLOOD PRESSURE.**

❑

NEW PUBLICATIONS

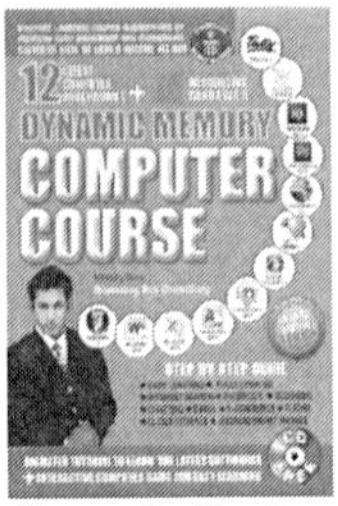

Biswaroop Roy Chowdhury
Dynamic Memory Computer Course (Updated & Revised)

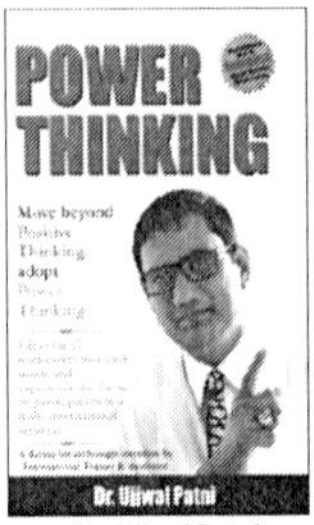

Dr. Ujjwal Patni
Power Thinking

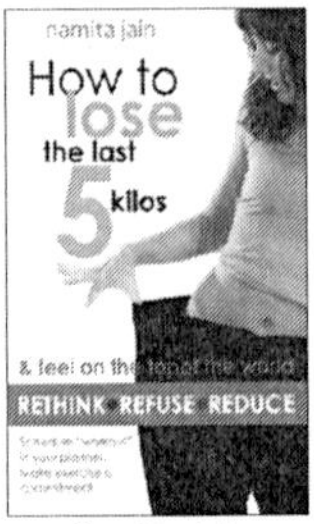

Namita Jain
How to Lose the last 5 Kilos

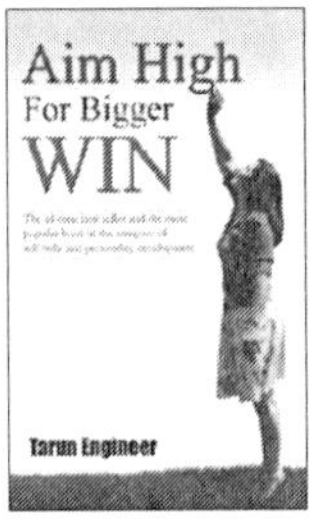

Tarun Engineer
Aim High For Bigger Win

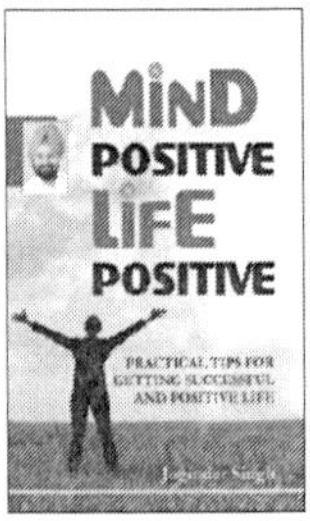

Joginder Singh
Mind Positive Life Positive

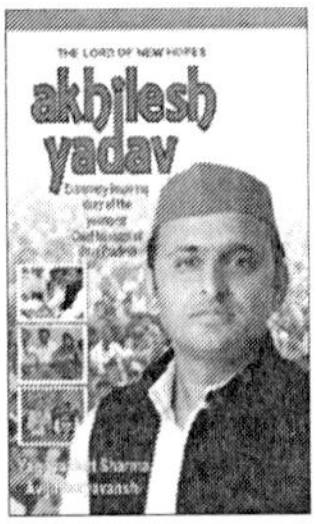

Yaggya Dutt Sharma
The Lord of New Hopes Akhilesh Yadav....

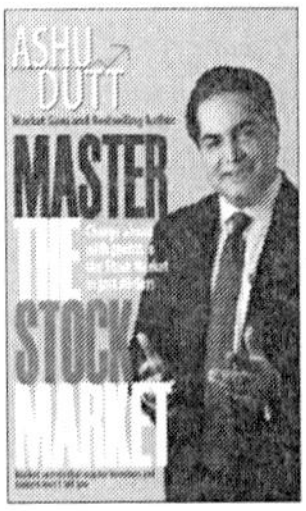

Ashu Dutt
Master the Stock Market

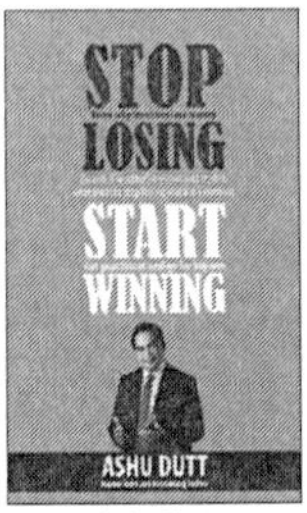

Ashu Dutt
Stop Losing Start Winning

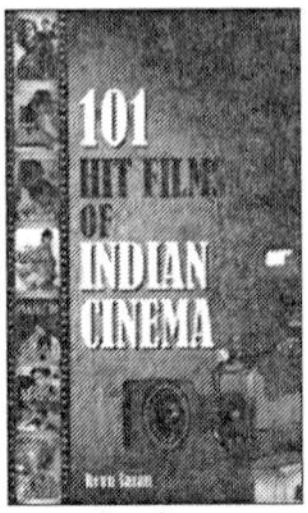

Renu Saran
101 Hit Films of Indian Cinema

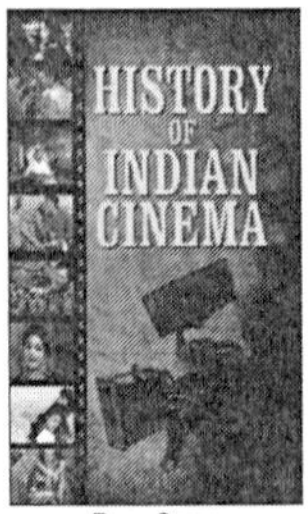

Renu Saran
History of Indian Cinema

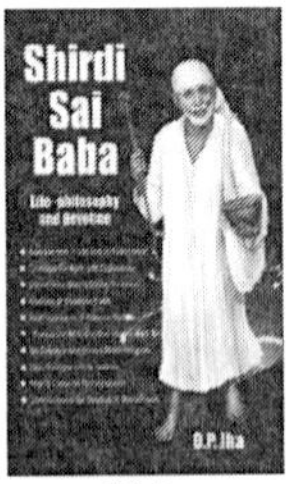

O.P. Jha
Shirdi Sai Baba: Life Philosophy and Devotion

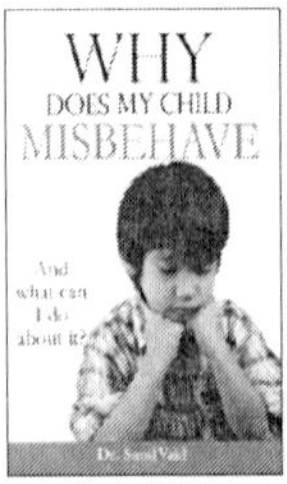

Dr. Sunil Vaid
Why Does My Child Misbehave

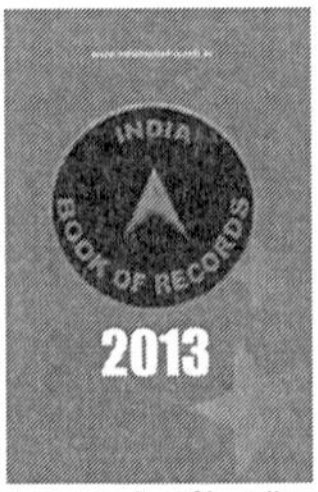

Biswaroop Roy Chowdhury
India Book of Records

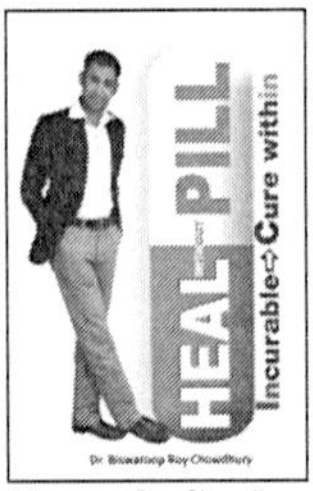

Biswaroop Roy Chowdhury
Heal Without Pill

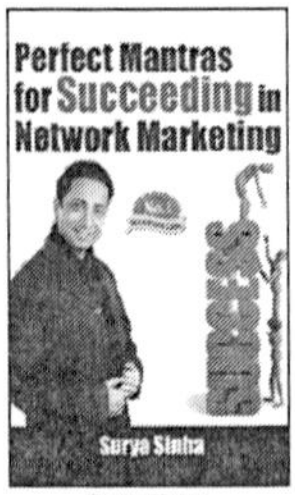

Surya Sinha
Perfect Mantras For Succeeding in Network Marketing

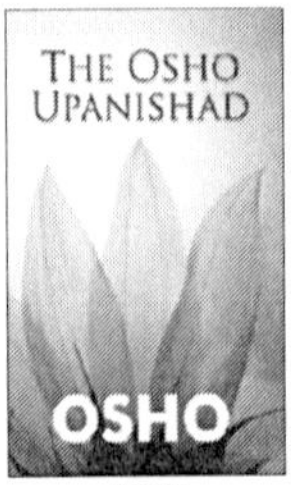

OSHO
The Osho Upanishad

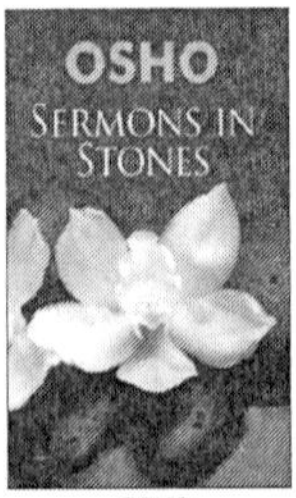

OSHO
Sermons in Stones

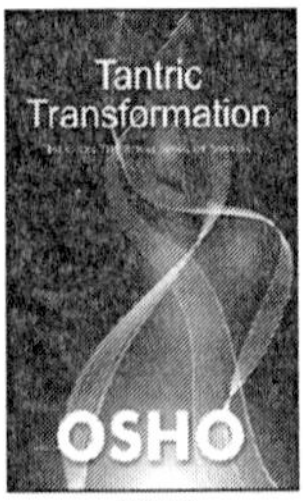

OSHO
Tantric Transformation

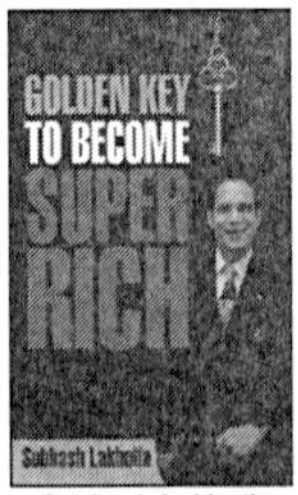

Subhash Lakhotia
Golden Key to Become Super Rich

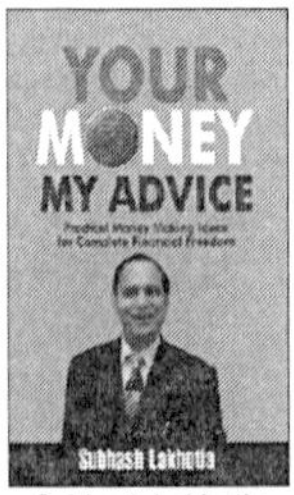

Subhash Lakhotia
Your Money My Advice

DIAMOND BOOKS X-30, Okhla Industrial Area, Phase-II New Delhi-110020
Tel : 011-40712200 email : sales@dpb.in
Shop online at www.diamondbook.in